Why Women Bury Men
THE LONGEVITY GAP IN CANADA

Why Women Bury Men

THE LONGEVITY GAP IN CANADA

BARBARA MURPHY

©2002, Barbara Murphy

All rights reserved. No part of this book may be reproduced, stored in a retrieval system or transmitted in any form or by any means without written permission from J. Gordon Shillingford Publishing Inc., except for brief excerpts used in critical reviews.

Cover design by Doowah Design Inc.
Cover photograph by Greg Klassen
Printed and bound in Canada

We acknowledge the financial assistance of the Manitoba Arts Council and
The Canada Council for the Arts for our publishing program.

Canadian Cataloguing in Publication Data

Murphy, Barbara
  Why women bury men: the longevity gap in Canada/
Barbara Murphy

ISBN 1-896239-91-9

  1. Longevity—Sex differences. 2. Aging—Sex Differences.
3. Health Behavior. I. Title.

RA776.75.M87 2002   612.6'8   C2002-902618-0

J. Gordon Shillingford Publishing
P.O. Box 86, 905 Corydon Avenue, Winnipeg, MB Canada R3M 3S3

To Paul, Kevin, and Jamie.

Acknowledgements

I want to acknowledge the work of a vast number of medical researchers in Canada and other countries whose findings form the basis for my contention that it is primarily lifestyles that keep men from living as long as women do. The absence of advocacy on this social issue is surprising, given the extent and substance of the research, but this is not really the responsibility of medical researchers whose job it is to provide their findings and leave social action to others.

In the course of showing the connection between lifestyles and specific diseases I have tried to give brief descriptions of the disease in question although I am not trained in medicine. I would like to thank medical professionals who read individual chapters for accuracy.: Dr. Nancy Carson, Director of Molecular Genetics Diagnostics Laboratory of Eastern Ontario Regional Genetics Program and Dr. Paul Hoskins, Medical Oncologist, B.C. Cancer Agency, also Associate Professor of Medicine, University of British Columbia. In describing diseases I have tried to use language that non-medical readers may find less technical than that used by professionals. If I have erred by oversimplifying, the responsibility is mine.

I would like to thank Jeannette Crosby for translation of articles in *Revue française sociologie*. I am also grateful for the service give by the staff of the Health Sciences library at the University of Ottawa and the MacOdrum Library at Carleton University.

Finally, Terry Gallagher has done it again. My thanks for her creative cover design.

Table of Contents

Chapter 1
Life Expectancies, Then and Now 11
Chapter 2
Female Biological Advantages 21
Chapter 3
Heart Disease and Lifestyles 33
Chapter 4
Cancer and Lifestyles 45
Chapter 5
Lung and Liver Diseases and Lifestyles 59
Chapter 6
The Risk-takers 69
Chapter 7
Mortality by Marital Status and Social Class 79
Chapter 8
Years of Life Lost 93
Chapter 9
Gender Differences, Widening and Narrowing ... 103
Chapter 10
Unknowns in the New Century 115
Endnotes 127
Selected Bibliography 135
Index 141

Chapter 1

Life Expectancies, Then and Now

Women live longer than men in every country of the world except Nepal. Less than 30 years ago in five undeveloped countries in South Asia men still outlived women, but the shift to longer female lives is now almost universal. Not only do women live longer than men, but they live up to 12 years longer—a gap of 11 years in Estonia and Lithuania, for example, and 12 years in Russia. In the world's population over 65 years of age there are at least 50 million more women than men.

In Canada the gap between male and female life expectancy, sometimes called the longevity gap, is six years. And because women tend to be two to three years younger than their husbands, most Canadian widows will be nine years on their own—a lonely life for the greater part of the elderly population. There are also economic implications: besides isolation and loneliness, widows experience dramatically changed day-to-day living conditions as a result of their reduced incomes. For society as a whole, there are added costs as single elderly women join the ranks of the poor.

We accept these social and economic consequences without much question. One of the greatest misconceptions among the general public is that a six-year shorter lifespan for men is beyond anyone's control. In fact, premature death for men is so readily taken for granted that it is not a pressing public health issue, not the subject of a national task force or royal commission, and not part of the concerns of any male advocacy organization. Instead it is considered an inevitable fact of life. Yet the six-year difference between men's and women's lifespans is not inevitable at all. Much of the difference is not laid down in any laws of nature or human biology. Many of the years can be attributed to men's lifestyles and their social roles, and among those non-biological influences there are many that can be changed.

For the most part, we choose our lifestyles. There may be less choice for those born into poverty or handicapped in some other way, but in general our behavioural characteristics are our own doing. In a lifetime of choices, as the following chapters will show, men tend to choose behaviour that shortens their lives. Why this is so is another question. Finding the evidence of self-destructive behaviour is easy; finding the reason is not.

One theory is that women value health more than men do, a theory with some support from research studies.[1] Years of child rearing and responsibility for ill family members may make women more attentive to health matters and more inclined to educate themselves about better health practices. It is an argument with some appeal in the implication that men are busier educating themselves about more important things that reach far beyond the home and family, the proper domain of women. On the other hand, lifestyle differences may have nothing to do with knowledge of health practices. Men may simply prefer to take chances with life, worrying less about unhealthy lifestyles, and leaving the future to look after itself.

These speculations presuppose that men *want* to live longer and are simply taking the wrong route. But perhaps men don't want to live longer at all. With an average life expectancy at birth of 75, most Canadian men will have been out of the labour force for several years by the time they die. The anticipation of many unproductive years (if they define productive as labour force participation) may offer little incentive to men to extend their lives. Unfortunately, such decisions are often made by younger men holding stereotypes of old age, views that are left behind as old age approaches. By then, however, it is too late. Medical research has shown again and again that it can be more than 20 years before lifestyle choices take their toll. Moreover, the anticipation of jobless years could apply to both sexes. There is no convincing reason why young and middle-aged men would fear unemployment in old age more than women do. Being out of the labour force may not represent as great a loss of status for women, but their increased labour force participation over the last half century makes this less likely as time goes by.

If loss of status is not the reason for fearing unemployment in old age, there is even less reason to fear loss of income. Statistics consistently show that older men are better off financially than older women. And financial circumstances do make a difference. In national surveys of retired people, income level is shown to be strongly associated with the level of satisfaction with life. There is also less reason for men than for women to fear poor health in old age. The irony is that, although their mortality rates are higher, men are more inclined to have illnesses that are short term (and indeed fatal). *If* they are still alive at an advanced age, they are less likely to have the non-fatal chronic or disabling illnesses that affect older women.[2] And as with income, good health is associated with happiness among older people.

Whatever their reasons, men choose lifestyles that shorten their lives and since choice is involved, a longevity gap of six years is not necessary nor predetermined by some unfortunate trick of nature. The kindest interpretation of the failure of men to connect lifestyle choices with lifespan is that they temporarily take leave of their senses while making these choices.

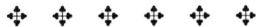

The advantage of women over men in lifespan is so clear in all developed countries today that we could mistakenly attribute it entirely to basic physical or biological differences between the sexes. But women did not always have this advantage. It is a phenomenon of the past two centuries and, since the basic biological characteristics of the human species have changed little during its long history, we have to look for other reasons for this relatively recent development. In fact, when we look further back than the nineteenth century we find the situation completely reversed. For over 75,000 years through primitive, nomadic, and early agricultural periods of human existence men lived longer than women.

All this should be placed in the context of the evolution of human lifespan in general throughout human history, without regard for gender differences. As social and economic development over thousands of years changed the way people lived, it also changed the way they died. The academic fields of both anthropology and demography are involved in the study of these changes. We owe our knowledge of early human lifespans to scientists in these two fields, especially to the lesser known discipline of palaeodemography which studies the skeletal finds of ancient cemeteries excavated by archaeologists.

These scientists have been able to determine the age at death of individual members of ancient populations by examining human skeletons. In particular, they study the degree of closure of the three main sutures of the skull, the internal structure of the long bones of the upper arms and thighs (their stage of development at time of death), and the surface condition of pelvic bones which also undergo developmental phases throughout life. From this information the lifespan of early man has been estimated with enough consistency that comparisons over time may be made.

Some 75,000 to 100,000 years ago, in what has been called the Old Stone Age, Neanderthal man lived in caves, used fire, and wore animal skins sewn with needles made from bones. It has been estimated from fossil remains in excavated cemeteries that members of these small populations (if they did not die as infants or young children, an extremely high probability) may have lived on average to the age of 35 or 36. Cro-Magnon man, the first modern man, came later, engaging in communal hunting and fishing, building boats and using harpoons. Lifespans of Cro-Magnon people were probably 43 years on average (again, if they escaped childhood mortality).

As ancient populations began to settle in villages, domesticate animals, and develop an early specialization of labour, lifespans gradually lengthened. In the Bronze and Iron Ages, extending across almost four centuries, life expectancy at birth continued to be short, given high infant mortality, but by the time of the Roman Empire those reaching 20 years of age could expect to live another 25 to 27 years, or to an age of roughly 46. Later, during the Middle Ages and the early period of feudalism, lifespans showed little change. Although economic conditions had improved since ancient times, primitive medical knowledge and sanitation were still factors affecting lifespan and, as a result, epidemics of plague and other communicable diseases often kept mortality high. Lifespan remained fairly static around 45 or 46 years.

Beginning with the seventeenth century written material on mortality is more available and is used as a source more frequently than cemetery excavations. The human lifespan changed slowly—those reaching adulthood could expect to live to 58 years of age by the middle of the nineteenth century, the beginning of a period called the demographic transition, and often more appropriately the demographic revolution.

Between the middle and the end of the nineteenth century the change in human lifespan was indeed revolutionary. Mortality rates dropped rapidly in the second half of the century as a result of social and economic changes and especially as a result of progress in medicine and hygiene. The discovery of the causes of various diseases, the introduction of effective vaccines, and the widespread application of new measures of public health were largely responsible. The decrease in infant mortality played an important part and continued to play a part through the first half of the twentieth century. Infant mortality in advanced countries of the world fell from an average of 150 per 1,000 births in 1900 to roughly 20 per 1,000 in 1950. Today infant mortality during the first year of life is 9 per 1,000 births in the United States and 6 per 1,000 in Canada, one of the lowest rates in the world, according to United Nations data.[3] With an infant mortality rate of less than one percent, lifespan expected at birth is now 78.5 years in Canada, more than twice that of prehistoric times and even twenty years longer than at mid-nineteenth century.

Throughout the thousands of years of slowly increasing human lifespans, men lived longer than women. As far back as the middle centuries of the Stone Age, men lived, on average, four years longer. In the Roman Era the gap was roughly the same, and throughout the Middle Ages men's lifespans continued to be longer than women's. By the nineteenth century, however, the situation reversed.

Two trends affecting lifespan began to develop alongside each other. Economic modernization raised standards of living, including the progress in medicine and hygiene mentioned earlier, in the more advanced countries of the world—western European and North American countries, as well as Australia and New Zealand. As a result, lifespans in general lengthened. At the same time, not everyone benefitted from the new longer lives to the same extent. Women began to live longer than men by roughly two years in Sweden, the Netherlands, and France—even before industrialization. By mid-nineteenth century most west European countries and North America were showing the same longevity advantage for women.

The shift was dramatic but the reason quite fundamental. The same social and economic changes that brought about revolutionary declines in mortality during the "demographic transition" also brought remarkable changes in the lives of women, especially changes in the physical demands made on them in earlier economies. In the traditional division of labour, women as far back as nomadic societies gathered food, hunted small prey, prepared meals, tanned animal skins, made clothing, produced pottery, and fetched water in addition to the annual rigours of pregnancy and childbirth. In agricultural societies they tended animals, churned butter, made soap, gathered fuel, fetched water, tilled fields, planted, harvested, winnowed, ground, baked, spun, wove, and sewed. *And* gave birth, nursed infants, and tended children. In the improved economic conditions of the early nineteenth century much of this burden on women disappeared. The result was that, as life expectancies for both men and women increased with a better standard of living, they increased to a greater extent for women.

Instead of simply catching up, however, women's lifespans surpassed men's by about two years, even though they both shared the same new economic conditions. It is generally believed that biological differences, with a disadvantage for men, explain the two-year gap in the early period of modernization. These innate male biological disadvantages had been around since the first appearance of modern man, but there had been little opportunity for them to surface when women were dying earlier from a heavier physical burden. As one team of longevity scholars explains, "In the course of history it was not the biological differences between the sexes that underwent modification, but rather the respective status of the sexes, and mortality conditions changed accordingly."[4] With economic modernization women lived a few years longer initially, then increased their lead dramatically as the twentieth century progressed. The advantage for women now stands at six years in Canada, a rather remarkable change in a single century after 750 centuries during which the longevity advantage belonged to men.

But a longer life was an empty victory. There was little to give cheer to widows in scientific articles that attributed their husbands' early deaths to the fact that men were indeed the weaker sex, their biological characteristics at the root of the problem. These biological characteristics, it was argued, were holding them back from the same benefits of economic modernization as women enjoyed. Today even the most bereaved widows are not likely to accept the "weaker sex" argument with all that it implies, that is, that men have apparently become weaker and weaker over the last century as the gap widened from two to six years. Without changes to basic human biology, biological differences between men and women fail to be convincing as the total cause of the gap. In fact, not only is biology far from being the total cause, it is only a small part of the cause. How men and women have reacted differently to economic modernization is the larger part—the styles of living they have used to adapt, the behaviours they have chosen as better living standards made life easier for everyone. These are the more important differences in explaining the longevity gap. They are worth analyzing in the search for answers.

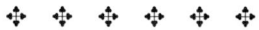

The most straightforward approach to exploring the gap between men and women in average lifespan is to look at the respective causes of their deaths. As an analytic approach, it has the advantage that all developed and many developing countries keep annual data on causes of death. Moreover, the analysis is simplified by the fact that the four or five leading causes of death in these countries comprise almost 75 percent of all deaths. In Canada, deaths from cancer, heart disease, stroke, respiratory diseases, and accidents, account for 79 percent of all deaths. Of course, if men and women were found to have similar mortality rates for each cause of death it would not be a productive approach, but this is far from the case.

The causes of death recorded in national statistics are gathered from death certificates filed by a doctor at the time of death. So they are the *immediate* cause of death. Fortunately considerable scientific research over the last century has isolated underlying or indirect causes behind each immediate cause. Research has shown that many people who die of a specific disease share similar biological characteristics or behavioural patterns or even social roles. The majority of people who die from cirrhosis of the liver, for example, have a pattern of immoderate alcohol consumption so while the immediate cause of death is liver disease, the indirect cause is alcohol consumption. In the same vein, the majority of people dying from lung cancer are smokers; the majority dying from accidents are people inclined toward hazardous behaviour.

Researchers, after finding male-female differences in mortality rates for the leading causes of death, have then looked to indirect causes for an explanation. If an indirect cause—a behaviour pattern or lifestyle—of a particular disease is found to be more common to men than to women, researchers propose that the behaviour explains the difference in male-female mortality rates for that disease. At the least the finding is considered a partial explanation. Without following specific individuals through longitudinal studies, proof is hard to come by. Of course, the stronger the similarity between male predominance among those dying from a particular disease and male predominance in a suspected behaviour pattern, the more we are likely to accept that the two are linked.

Throughout the developed world, according to United Nations statistics, the leading causes of death are cardiovascular disease, cancer, respiratory diseases, and accidents. For every leading cause of death, men have higher mortality rates than women. In Canada, men are almost twice as likely to die of heart and respiratory diseases, twice as likely to die of lung cancer, and two and a half times as likely to die as a result of accidents or violence than women.[5] If we can explain these heavy odds against men, we can go a long way to explaining why women live longer. The chapters that follow will look for these explanations in the current findings of longevity researchers who examine the indirect causes, or the risk factors, of the leading causes of death.

Dividing up the six-year longevity gap into precise parts that can be attributed to specific causes has not been attempted by many researchers. It has not been attempted for obvious reasons—segregating such causes from a whole range of other developments that happen at the same time in modern countries is almost impossible. Still, where research scientists have been strongly convinced of the relative contribution made by certain indirect causes of death, their findings are presented.

At the base of the six years are roughly two years attributed to biological differences between men and women that appear to favour women. These differences—to be covered in the following chapter—may be intriguing, but they fail to explain in full why the longevity gap has grown over two centuries while biological differences have stayed the same.

CHAPTER 2

Female Biological Advantages

Although few medical researchers have been precise in estimating the portion of the longevity gap that can be attributed to biological differences, the estimates that can be found attribute only a small portion. In fairness, it appears that these rare attempts are more for the purpose of underlining the importance of social and behavioural factors in longevity which were ignored for a good part of the past century.

Demographer Roland Pressat points out that evidence of biological differences can be found in the higher mortality of male infants compared to female infants during the first year of life, a period when behavioural and social factors have not had an opportunity to influence sex differences. He maintains that these innate biological differences result in a moderate difference of about two years between the lifespans of men and women.[6] While not volunteering a specific proportion, gerontologist Lois Verbrugge contends that biological factors rank last after lifestyles, social roles, and health practices in sex differences in mortality. Overall, the impact of biological factors, she believes, is "quite small over the life course."[7]

Ingrid Waldron, a geneticist, is reluctant to estimate the size of the contribution of biological factors. She argues that methodological difficulties make precise estimation impossible. In addition, the effects of biological factors vary depending on environmental conditions. She believes, however, that while lower infant mortality for females may be due primarily to biological factors, these factors may not play such a large role throughout the rest of life. Instead, widespread social and cultural influences on male behaviour as compared to female behaviour may be the primary cause of the differences in their mortality.[8]

Whatever portion of the gender gap can be attributed to biological factors, much of the evidence is still under study. Biology, especially the field of genetics, is a fast-moving science these days, and new discoveries are made almost weekly. The remainder of this chapter considers the evidence to date of the biological contribution.

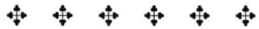

For the portion of the gender gap that may be attributed to biological differences between men and women there are generally four areas where evidence has increasingly shown a contribution. Among the four, the most frequently described as conclusive is the role of sex hormones.

Over the past 20 years several studies have shown that the female sex hormone, estrogen, may provide a protective effect for women against heart disease, the leading cause of death in Canada and throughout the world. The studies have been based on measures of levels of cholesterol, a known contributor to constriction of the arteries. The risk of heart disease rises with advancing age for both sexes, but the mortality rate for women lags approximately a decade behind that of men throughout the entire lifespan. In Canada, men are almost twice as likely as women to die from this cause alone.

Ranking as the leading cause of death, heart disease has been the subject of considerable study in the last half of the twentieth century. Narrowing of the arteries, the chief culprit, is known to be strongly associated with cholesterol, a fatty or oil-like substance that may be deposited (if in excess) in the walls of the aorta and its major branches including the coronary arteries, obstructing the smooth passage of blood. Two kinds of cholesterol play a part. High-density lipoprotein (HDL) cholesterol, low levels of which are the most powerful risk factor for heart disease, is often called the good cholesterol. When HDL cholesterol levels are high, the risk of heart disease is low. Low-density lipoprotein (LDL) cholesterol is the bad cholesterol. When LDL levels are high, so too is the risk of heart disease.

Interestingly the levels of bad cholesterol rise for both sexes from puberty on, but they rise faster and stay higher in men until middle age, accounting in part for their higher risk of heart disease. The situation changes, however, at the female menopause, when estrogen levels in women drop. At that time their bad cholesterol levels increase significantly, matching and exceeding levels for men of the same age and continuing to do so for the remainder of life. These findings were the first clue to a role for estrogen in modulating and balancing cholesterol levels.[9]

The mechanisms by which estrogen affects cholesterol levels favourably are not clear. The bad cholesterol (LDL) undergoes a process of oxidation which makes a major contribution to narrowing of the arteries. It has been suggested by biologist Tessa Pollard, however, that estrogen appears to inhibit that process, dilating the blood vessels and preventing constriction.[10]

On the strength of natural estrogen's benefits, many post-menopausal women over the past decade have received exogenous estrogen to protect against heart disease. To reduce the risk of cancer, progestins were added to the estrogen in what has been called hormonal replacement therapy. The most recent studies have found, however, that the protective effects of estrogen related to the heart may be counteracted by progestin. For example, progestin may act to block estrogen's beneficial effect on lipoproteins and may also reduce its vasodilator effect. As a result, hormone replacement therapy has provided no protection against heart disease for women and has, in fact, increased the risk.

It is also not clear whether estrogen has any part in the female advantage of higher levels of good cholesterol (HDL) over the lifespan. There is no drop in HDL cholesterol during or after menopause, a drop that would indicate a connection. The advantage is more likely due to hormonal effects on male HDL that keep it low. Biologists suggest this trend may be attributed to the effect of the male sex hormone, androgen, in keeping male HDL levels lower, given the continued secretion of androgen throughout adult life.[11]

All this points to an increasingly evident positive role for female sex hormones in the longevity gap and a less important negative role for male sex hormones. Estrogen protects women against heart disease, while androgen, the male sex hormone, plays a lesser role but still may be responsible for making men more vulnerable. Besides their effects on cholesterol, sex hormones may also play a role, though a lesser one, in male-female differences in immune response and in the handling of stress, two other areas of female biological advantage to be covered in this chapter.

❖ ❖ ❖ ❖ ❖ ❖

A second area biologists consider important in male-female longevity differences is the human immune function.

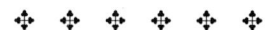

There appears to be general agreement that this function in humans diminishes with age. The increase in cancer and infectious diseases in elderly people are often attributed to this declining level. As people age, their antibody production goes down, and with it, their protection against disease. At the same time it appears that women are less affected by this decline in immune function; this could contribute to the gender gap in longevity. Studies of the white blood cells that produce antibodies show less decline in cell numbers for women than for men as they grow older. In effect, their immune systems remain better preserved.[12]

While this accounts for their immunity advantage in later years, females also demonstrate greater immune responses than males earlier in life. Animal studies illustrate the difference. In one study with young mice, skin grafts were rejected by more female mice (55 percent) than by males (28 percent).[13] Other animal studies have shown similar evidence of greater immune activity among females, including more tumour resistance.

The reasons for greater female immunity are not clear, but several theories exist. Levels of immunoglobulin M (IgM), an antibody in human blood cells, have been studied in an attempt to find the answer. Serum samples taken from over 400 individuals in an American study in Virginia showed that IgM concentrations are higher in females than males. Both children and adults were included. In another study of over 800 individuals in California, the same significant difference was found between male and female levels of IgM.[14]

The Virginia study also found a strong link between the IgM concentrations of parents and their offspring, pointing to a genetic basis for immunoglobulin; that is, a gene carried on the human X chromosome (the female sex chromosome) may affect immunoglobulin concentration and ultimately give survival advantage. It appears that the X chromosome carries one or more genes that influence IgM production. Since female cells contain two X chromosomes compared to the single X chromosome in male cells, this may give an advantage to females in immunoglobulin level.[15] There are other possibilities for the X chromosome in female longevity. The whole genetic argument is covered in the next section.

Besides a possible genetic influence on the stronger immune system of females there may also be a role for sex hormones. In addition to their capacity to handle cholesterol and provide a certain amount of protection against heart disease as discussed earlier, sex hormones may modulate other immune responses. It has been found that male sex hormones in particular can have a deleterious effect. When female mice are treated with male sex hormones, their production of specific antibodies is reduced. In contrast, when male mice are castrated (depriving them of testosterone), their production of these antibodies is increased.[16] These disadvantages for men, of course, become advantages for women in their comparative mortality rates.

It appears that women's immune systems are stronger for both genetic and hormonal reasons. They have higher levels of one of the major immunoglobulins and they lose fewer important antibodies as they age. This heightened immune activity for females may contribute to their greater longevity, while men's immune activity may be weakened by male sex hormones, making the longevity gap even wider.

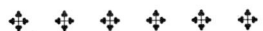

Besides the contribution of human hormonal and immune systems, the human genome may contribute to the longevity gap. Scientists often attribute women's longer lifespan to an innate vulnerability in men by virtue of their possession of only one X chromosome.

It is a well known biological fact that female mammals of all species have two X chromosomes while males have an X chromosome and a Y chromosome. In females one X chromosome is derived from the mother and one from the father; in males the X chromosome is derived from the mother and the Y chromosome from the father. Called the sex chromosomes because they determine the sex of the human child, the pair of Xs or the X and Y set occur in every cell of the body along with 44 other chromosomes that are unrelated to sex. The 44 non-sex chromosomes are actually 22 pairs and they are similar in men and women.

The X chromosome in both males and females contains many genes involved in vital functions; for example, genes related to blood clotting, muscle function, protection against oxidative damage, DNA synthesis, and immune response. Women have two sets of these genes to choose from, while men have only a single copy. There is the potential, therefore, for essential functions that map to the X chromosome to give greater longevity to the female.

In addition, there is a further sex chromosome advantage for females. A process early in female development inactivates one of the two X chromosomes in each cell of the female organism. Geneticists explain that this process, called dosage compensation, occurs in order to achieve the same amount of X linked genes in women as available to men with only one X chromosome. Because some cells have the maternal X chromosome active after the inactivation process and others have the paternal X active, the female cell system has been called a mosaic, and biologists frequently refer to the mosaic nature of the female. One might expect this process, which takes away the functioning of one X chromosome, to reduce the advantage for women, but it appears to have one or two surprising benefits. Defective genes in some cells, perhaps defects that may cause certain diseases, can be compensated by neighbouring cells where the other X chromosome is active and has an intact non-defective gene. Clearly this compensation cannot take place in male cells with only one X chromosome.

As cells proliferate in the female mosaic, a selection process also appears to take place, often adaptive. In other words, cells with defective genes may be selected against. The organism may instead select those cells with the X chromosome containing genes most likely to contribute to optimum development. Indeed, selection would be in the direction of the most balanced composition of chromosomes possible. Such cell selection resulting in better functioning of the organism can only occur in females and could be another reason for their greater longevity.[17]

A genetic benefit, therefore, appears to be in play for women's longer lifespans by their possession of two X chromosomes and a complex process of selection that is not available to men.

✤ ✤ ✤ ✤ ✤ ✤

A fourth area where biological differences may play a role in the longevity gap is stress. It has been popular to attribute the greater longevity of women in modern countries to the effects of occupational stress on men. Yet it is now recognized that both men and women are exposed to daily stressful experiences, though these experiences may be of a different nature. And while both men and women are exposed, it appears that biology has not given men a break on the impact of stress.

Put simply, stress is a perception of excessive demands that any man or woman feels they are unable to meet or manage. Faced with stress the human body behaves as it did earlier in our evolutionary history with a "fight or flight" response, even if such a response is no longer appropriate. In this response the main so-called "stress hormones," adrenaline and cortisol, are secreted as a measure to adapt the body to the new demand.

The secretion of adrenaline stimulates the release of nutritive material that can be used to provide immediate sources of energy. Glucose and fats would be among those released. But if modern man no longer fights or flees, these energy sources are not required, and fatty acids in particular may simply be added to other fats that raise cholesterol levels. Indirectly, then, adrenaline contributes to one of the main risk factors for heart disease.[18]

There are two other problems related to adrenaline. It affects cell fragments called platelets, whose function in the bloodstream is the clotting of blood. The presence of adrenaline causes these fragments to become more cohesive in the arteries which, in turn, raises the risk of clot formation leading to a heart attack or stroke. Adrenaline is also involved in regulating blood pressure. Continued stress and the adrenaline secreted to adapt the body to it may keep blood pressure elevated, with the obvious risk of sustained hypertension, damage to the arterial walls, and the narrowing of arteries that leads to heart disease.

With this fallout from adrenaline, it is of interest that men appear to show greater adrenaline response than women in stress situations. This is another instance where estrogen may provide women with protection not available to men. Evidence that post-menopausal women lose this apparent protection against the effects of high levels of adrenaline has led researchers to this conclusion. And conversely, post-menopausal women who undergo estrogen replacement therapy have been found to show blunted adrenaline responses to stress compared to post-menopausal women without estrogen replacement.[19]

So the sex hormone, estrogen, can provide some protection against the effects of the stress hormone, adrenaline. Presumably its protection is through its capacity to modulate and balance cholesterol levels as we have seen earlier, and—in the case of stress—these cholesterol levels can become unbalanced by the unnecessary fatty acids released into the arteries by adrenaline. Without estrogen, men show a greater adrenaline response to stress and a greater risk of heart disease.

Studies have also shown that, in the face of stress, men exhibit higher systolic blood pressure changes than women do. In tests the difference between men and women has been significant.[20] While adrenaline has effects on the levels of everyone's blood pressure, often bad effects, it is apparent from these studies that women are not affected as strongly as men. The reasons for this finding are still not known.

Stress, adrenaline, increased fats in the body, and elevated blood pressure are all tied together and contribute to greater risks for men for heart disease or stroke. Estrogen may be a partial explanation for the better responses of women to stress, but it is clearly not the total explanation. In addition to biological responses, behavioural responses to stress, to be discussed in a later chapter, may also play a role.

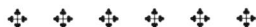

Women live longer than men, and there are both biological and behavioural explanations for this phenomenon in modernized countries. Evidence has been provided in this chapter to show that there are at least four biological areas that could account for a female longevity advantage. It is not always possible, however, to separate the two kinds of explanations. In some instances, biological factors may not directly affect the longevity gap between men and women. They may instead have an indirect effect by becoming a part of human culture and influencing social behaviour and social roles long past the time when the original biological cause has ceased to be relevant.

The most obvious of these indirect influences is the inherent sex differences in reproductive function in human society, a biological fact of hundreds of thousands of years that has had indirect effects in the last century that may contribute to some of the longevity gap.

An original effect of the different reproductive roles was that throughout early history, women—the only ones able to bear and nurse children—were assigned the primary responsibility for the care of children. With this responsibility they were unable to take on dangerous tasks or other work that was incompatible with child care. These tasks were instead assigned to men. Over centuries the rearing of young boys has included preparing them to take part in the dangerous activities associated with this role for men. It is still part of the socializing of children today.

The indirect consequence of this cultural development has been that men are more inclined toward risk-taking behaviour than women, a tendency that is reflected in their high rate of mortality due to accidents. In Canada fatal accidents were the fourth leading cause of death in 1997 (after cardiovascular diseases, cancer, and respiratory diseases), and the accident mortality rate for men was two and a half times that of women. This is also the average male-female ratio for all reporting countries of the world, according to United Nations figures.

To the extent that a good percentage of fatal accidents, especially motor vehicle accidents, are alcohol-related (an estimated 48 percent in Canada), the lower mortality rates for women could similarly be traced back to their reproductive role. Historically, women have been under social pressure to refrain from heavy drinking because of their child care responsibilities and, as a result, only in the last century did it become acceptable for women to drink. Today they are still less likely to drink than men. Among regular drinkers in Canada, that is, drinkers who consume one or more alcoholic drinks per month, the proportion of males is one and a half times the proportion of females.

Another biological factor may have an indirect effect on male-female differences in fatal accidents. The male sex hormone may be responsible for the generally accepted observation that men are more aggressive than women. It is a well known fact that, in many non-human mammals, males demonstrate more fighting behaviour than females. Early experiments with mammals showed that this male trait was determined by levels of the male hormone, androgen. Male rats, for instance, engage in spontaneous fighting around the time of puberty, but when castrated in laboratory experiments their aggressive behaviour diminished. However, injections of testosterone, the principal male steroid hormone, restored their readiness to fight.[21] Over the years similar results have been found. Experiments with mice also connected aggressive behaviour with testosterone. Newborn *female* mice, receiving injections of testosterone in experimental studies, have exhibited the same fighting behaviour as male mice. Hamsters treated with testosterone have responded in the same way.²² Studies have also looked at aggression in rhesus monkeys and found that aggressive behaviour was related to higher levels of testosterone.

Just as with rats, mice, hamsters, and monkeys, humans also demonstrate a sex difference in aggressive behaviour. Whether the aggressiveness of human males is related to the male sex hormone as it is with other mammals has not been proven. Studies have shown that a relationship exists but, until they are replicated satisfactorily, the issue is still up in the air.

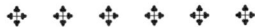

Biologists suggest that these four areas—sex hormones, the immune function, sex chromosome differences, and stress—provide some of the answer to why women live longer than men. In addition, there have been indirect effects of the different reproductive roles of men and women which can be found in cultural and behavioural influences on certain diseases and ultimately on mortality.

Before leaving the subject of biological factors, it is interesting to consider what purpose for the survival of the human species is served by innate biological differences that translate into greater longevity for women. The average longevity for a species in general, that is longevity for both sexes, is known to include the reproductive years for obvious reasons of species survival through reproduction. In humans, unlike many non-human species, average longevity goes well past the reproductive years to accommodate the long period of dependency of the human young. It is not only the length of the human lifespan that has accommodated survival needs. It has also been suggested that the higher concentrations of immunoglobulin M antibodies in women (believed to be affected by genes carried by the X chromosome) may originally have been of evolutionary importance in maternal survival during the long human gestation period and the extended immaturity of the young.²³ The protection provided by female sex hormones up to the menopause may have been just as important. There seems to have been some sense of purpose to all this. Today with roughly 40 percent of the life cycle beyond the reproductive years, it is easy to lose sight of these origins. Instead we are more likely to question the purpose of innate biological differences between men and women that result in the end in an elderly population substantially made up of women.

CHAPTER 3

Heart Disease and Lifestyles

Ischemic heart disease is the leading cause of death in developed countries of the world, and men are twice as likely as women to die of it. According to United Nations statistics, ischemic heart disease, which until recently was known as coronary heart disease, was the single leading cause in the 1990s in Canada, United States, United Kingdom, France, Germany, Italy, Netherlands, Norway, Sweden, Australia and New Zealand.[24]

In Canada over 79,000 individuals died of diseases of the circulatory system in 1997, 77 percent of whom died of heart disease.[25] Since men are twice as likely as women to die from heart disease, it accounts for roughly one-third of the longevity gap between men and women, or two years of the six-year gap. Male-female differences in lung cancer mortality, by comparison, account for less than a year.[26]

The importance of heart disease, of course, is due to the importance of the body's circulatory system to life itself. The whole system of blood pumping through arteries, capillaries, and veins provides the body with vital nutrients and oxygen. But the heart, the pumping organ of the body, can only do its job if the flow of blood is unobstructed. With the constant passage of blood through the arteries, thickening of the artery walls can take place and the passageways narrow. The process of thickening of the innermost portion of the artery, called atherosclerosis, begins when natural fatty substances and calcium become deposited in the artery wall. The inside diameter of the passageway narrows, and the resulting buildup, called a plaque, can make it difficult for blood to pass through.

Besides the contribution of fatty substances or cholesterol to the buildup of plaques, it is known that high blood pressure also contributes to atherosclerosis by damaging arterial walls. With this damage, both large and small arteries become scarred, hardened, and less elastic, a process that sometimes occurs with age in any event, but clearly does not benefit from the additional acceleration it receives from high blood pressure.

The body's blood circulating system, with its efficiency and self-regulation, is a remarkable achievement of nature. It is a humbling reality that the human brain played no part in its invention. Nonetheless, the size and complexity of the human brain that separates us from other living species has allowed us to understand how this inner system works. Instead of being in awe, however, instead of prizing this gift of nature, we have found many ways to make a highly efficient circulatory system less efficient.

Diseases of the heart do not develop as an inevitable consequence of aging. As one medical researcher states, "Coronary heart disease can be seen as a disorder of lifestyle, and many of its etiologic agents are potentially modifiable."[27] Besides physiological risk factors like high blood pressure and elevated blood cholesterol levels, human behaviours that contribute to the acceleration of atherosclerosis are also considered risk factors for heart disease. It is widely accepted that these include smoking, stress, poor diet, lack of exercise, and psychological factors such as anxiety and hostility. It may be useful, if not particularly cheerful, to look at each of these contributing factors in turn.

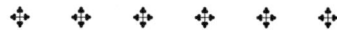

Smoking is a classic risk factor for heart disease in both men and women. Smokers are almost twice as likely as non-smokers to acquire ischemic heart disease with the risk directly related to the number of cigarettes smoked daily and the tar and nicotine content of the cigarette.[28]

The World Health Organization estimates that there are about 1.1 billion daily smokers in the world, equivalent to one-third of all persons aged 15 years or over. Although the proportion of male smokers in developed countries has dropped over the past 25 years, World Health Organization figures show that worldwide they still represent 73 percent of all smokers. It has been estimated that by the end of the twentieth century, smoking was responsible for 1.9 million deaths in developed countries, the large majority of them male deaths.[29]

In Canada the proportion of men among all smokers is 53 percent, more than the proportion of men in the general population. Almost 400,000 more men than women smoke. The good news is that since 1985 the number of Canadian smokers has declined by 15 percent. Within this general decline men took an earlier start than women, their smoking prevalence having peaked in the 1960s, while smoking prevalence for women did not peak until a decade later. Despite this head start for men, however, almost 27 percent of men still smoke compared to 23 percent of women.[30]

There are interesting variations in smoking prevalence by province, especially as related to sex differences. In Newfoundland, P.E.I., Nova Scotia, Quebec, and Alberta the percentage of male smokers is higher than the national average. In New Brunswick the percentage of female smokers is slightly higher than the percentage for males. In Ontario and B.C. the percentage of smokers is lower than the national average in total and for males and females. In almost all provinces the percentage of teenage females who smoke is greater than the percentage of teenage males who smoke, a trend that reverses by the age of twenty.

With roughly 6 million Canadians smoking daily, it might be interesting to review how this popular behaviour pattern affects the functioning of their cardiovascular systems.

The connection between smoking and the body's blood coagulation system has been shown in many studies.[31] Blood platelets, described earlier in considering the various effects of stress, are cell fragments whose function is the clotting of blood. Along with red and white blood cells they flow through the circulating system and, if all goes well, they will perform their function without mishap. Unfortunately a number of factors can cause platelets to stick together instead of moving in the bloodstream independently. When they stick together (or "aggregate") they can increase the damage to artery walls that may have already started in the form of lesions.

Smoking is one of the factors that causes the aggregation of platelets by a process that is not yet clear. An iron-containing substance found in tobacco leaves is suspected. When tobacco smoke is inhaled, the substance may find its way into the circulating blood where it can cause the aggregation of platelets.[32] Sticking to each other and sticking to damaged areas of artery walls, platelets may accelerate the process of atherosclerosis, leading to obstruction in the arteries and eventually blood clotting, or thrombosis.

Smoking, or specifically the nicotine in tobacco, also has an impact on the cardiovascular system by way of the nervous system.[33] Nicotine stimulates the sympathetic nerve cells, which in turn release certain hormones (the catecholamine or stress hormones) into the bloodstream. This release of stress hormones into the bloodstream is the same process set in motion by the human body and the bodies of most mammals when they respond to stress. It may be this process that causes many smokers to feel that their performance of a challenging task is improved by smoking.

As with the body's normal stress response, however, that sudden rush of energy is where the good part of the story ends. As we have seen with prolonged stress response, adrenaline and other catecholamine hormones increase both blood pressure and heart rate, and if these reactions occur repeatedly in daily life, as they do with smoking, they may increase the risk of coronary heart disease.

The release of catecholamine hormones into the bloodstream, caused by nicotine, can cause other damage as well. The catecholamines raise the level of free fatty acids in the blood, wreaking further damage on the plaques that are already narrowing the arteries. And this can occur independently of the damage caused by the aggregation of platelets.[34] The arteries, therefore, get a double whammy from smoking. Small wonder that it is a major risk factor for heart disease.

With these effects on the body's nervous system and

cardiovascular function, smoking is clearly harmful to both men and women. That twice as many men as women die of heart disease is to a large extent due to the fact that more men than women smoke. When we look for reasons for the widening gap between male and female life expectancies from the early to the late twentieth century, smoking heads the list. As smoking in general increased in the last hundred years and the mortality rates for smokers became dramatically higher compared to non-smokers, the fact that a much higher proportion of men smoked than women had the inevitable outcome. Scientists have attributed as much as 75 percent of the widening longevity gap during that period to smoking.[35]

It is easier to explain why men who smoke are more likely to die of heart disease than it is to explain why men are more likely to smoke in the first place. There are cultural reasons, some suggested in the last chapter, that attribute more risk-taking behaviour to men by virtue of their historical role in taking on dangerous tasks. It is not too far a stretch of logic to see smoking as a modern version of risk-taking. Medical researcher David Smith goes further, calling it self-destructive behaviour, along with alcohol abuse, and identifying both as contributors to the longevity gap between men and women.[36] It is possible as well that social pressures of the past against women smoking were also partly responsible for a greater number of male smokers. It is certainly true that as these pressures relaxed, women took up smoking in increasing numbers.

As smoking prevalence declined in the last part of the twentieth century, mortality rates for heart disease also declined during the same period, underlining the connection between the two and holding out some hope that, with the decline in a male-dominated cause of death, the longevity gap may narrow.

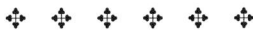

It has always been popular to attribute the difference in life expectancy between men and women to stress. In particular, the higher rate of male mortality due to heart disease was linked for the most part with greater stress in men's daily lives right up until the beginning of the last quarter of the twentieth century when the data on smoking started to come in. As smoking prevalence decreases in developed countries, stress may again become one of the major social risk factors for heart disease but for now, male-female differences in stress exposure are far from clear.

Before looking at social or non-biological factors related to stress, it is worth recalling that there are biological differences between men and women in their stress responses. The secretion of adrenaline that helps our bodies meet the demands of stress can be harmful to the circulatory system by raising blood pressure and cholesterol levels, both of which contribute to thickening or damaging the arteries. Adrenaline and other catecholamine hormones also make blood platelets more cohesive, leading to clot formation or thrombosis. With research evidence that men show greater adrenaline response to stress, the odds are they will experience more of these harmful effects. The differences between male and female responses may not be large in single exposures to stress, but if modern life presents daily stressful situations the small differences add up. Such was the case in the twentieth century as economic modernization and urbanization brought a new kind of occupational stress. Given the almost full labour force participation of men compared to the small participation of women in the first two-thirds of the century, occupational stress clearly had a greater impact on men.

The body's response to stress, while involving both the hormonal system and the nervous system, has its beginning with psychological reactions, that is, how we perceive the demands made on us. So important is individual perception that we sometimes fail to see why another person experiences stress in a situation we may not consider stressful. This is particularly true with occupational stress. Initial research into this kind of stress dealt with men in management positions, on the assumption that the competitiveness of modern business took its toll on high-powered management decision-makers. Research spread to the study of other occupations and finally to the study of job characteristics that could apply to any job, regardless of its label. This kind of research proved more fruitful since it took into account excessive workloads and the ability of a worker to control the nature of his or her job, that is, its speed and other working conditions. These conditions could apply to any job, managerial, blue-collar, or service.

A low level of control over one's job and a high workload turned out to be a combination that led to stress.[37] Studies of workers on assembly lines, for instance, showed that workers whose work pace was controlled by the speed of the assembly line had higher levels of catecholamine hormone excretion than workers who were able to pace their own activities. Jobs with high demand and low control over working conditions were the subject of subsequent studies, and all showed that heart disease was more prevalent among workers holding such jobs than those with lower work demands and greater control. Interestingly, high demand and low control jobs included such a variety as waiter or waitress, telephone operator, mail worker, and fireman, all associated with increased coronary heart disease risk. In contrast, low demand and high decision control jobs were, among others, forester, dentist, and natural scientist with lower risks for heart disease. Managers tended to be in high demand jobs, but stress levels were lower due to their greater control over decision-making.

With more men than women in the labour force, studies that demonstrated the negative effects of occupational stress on heart disease explained part of the higher mortality of men from that cause. But as women entered the labour force in greater numbers in the last third of the twentieth century, occupational stress findings became more relevant for women. It became clear that the majority of women were in low-paid jobs where workload demand was high and control over working conditions low. Still, men continued to maintain higher mortality rates.

A glimmer of change came by the 1980s when growth in the longevity gap between men and women levelled off and decreased slightly. Looking for answers, researchers began to study the relationship between these changes and the increase of women in the work force. Would greater female mortality follow? The answers have been interesting, especially as research has expanded into both on-the-job and off-the-job stresses for women in their new multiple roles. These will be the subject of a later chapter. Today, despite a new high of 69 percent female labour force participation,[38] men are still almost twice as likely as women to die of heart disease.

Somewhat related to the effects of stress on heart disease were the findings some years ago that certain behaviour characteristics made up a so-called coronary-prone personality. The Type A behaviour pattern that became the focus of several studies was characterized by intense striving for achievement, competitiveness, easily provoked impatience, time urgency, abruptness of gesture and speech, overcommitment to job, and excesses of drive and hostility.[39] Type A behaviour was shown to be closely related to subsequent heart disease and was more commonly found in men than in women.

By the 1980s further studies began to show less connection between Type A behaviour and heart disease. It became evident that not all of the behaviours listed in the Type A pattern contributed equally to coronary risk. Researchers began to study them separately, and what emerged was a stronger association between heart disease and three characteristics: hostility (or a tendency to respond to frustration with feelings of anger or irritation), unwillingness or inability to express anger outwardly, and vigorous speech. To a great extent these parts of Type A behaviour have replaced the total group of Type A behaviour characteristics in predicting coronary heart disease, but whether the three parts are also more prevalent among men is not clear.

There is a final link with stress in considering risk factors for heart disease. While both stress and smoking share some common physiological responses (increased heart rate and increased circulation of catecholamines), some research shows that the responses are additive and, in fact, that the two risk factors have a complex relationship, interacting to increase the risk of heart disease. Smoking has been shown to reduce a smoker's feelings of anxiety, whether the feelings are appropriate or inappropriate, and in doing so may lead the smoker to extended attempts to cope with stressful tasks. The prolonged coping, of course, means prolonged exposure to stress and its inevitable harmful effects.[40] This aspect of the smoking-stress relationship—smoking to reduce stress while actually prolonging it—has been called the nicotine paradox. To the extent that a greater percentage of men are smokers, the nicotine paradox could contribute to their greater mortality from heart disease.

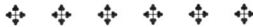

Lack of exercise and poor diet are also associated with heart disease. The differences between men and women in these two risk factors, however, appears to make only a minor contribution to the gap in their mortality rates.

In reviewing mortality levels across the world, the United Nations points out that in most developed market-economy countries, the physical activity of populations declined just as mortality fell. This was especially true as occupations shifted out of farming and other primary sectors in the twentieth century. This decline suggests that physical activity may not be a major determinant of a longer life. Yet studies looking at the connection between regular exercise during leisure time and heart health all demonstrate that mortality risks are lower among persons who exercise regularly. Regular physical activity can reduce body weight, improve serum cholesterol levels, and improve blood pressure.

In Canada national population health surveys, now carried out every two years, can track the risk of heart disease with some accuracy. The 1996-97 survey indicated that those who were inactive in their leisure time (but in good health) in 1994-95 had five times the odds of developing heart disease over the next two years as did moderately active or active people.[41] Roughly 60 percent of Canadian adults exercised three or more times weekly in 1998-99, a modest national performance shared equally by both men and women.

Similarly there are few studies showing significant male-female differences in the quality of diet. In fact, there is not a great deal of evidence that the general populations of many developed countries have acted on the strong evidence linking high levels of saturated fat intake (fat mainly of animal origin) with serum cholesterol levels and the incidence of heart disease. United Nations studies highlight the fact that countries that have adopted diets richer in fruits and vegetables and with a lower content of meat products and other sources of saturated fat have marked reductions in mortality.

While Canadian men and women appear to rank equally on exercise frequency and appropriate diet, there are differences in their tendencies to be overweight, a common risk factor for high blood pressure and heart disease. Over 59 percent of Canadian men between the ages of 15 and 65 are overweight compared to 37 percent of women.[42] In other words, a greater proportion of men are eating more calories than they need. If the average daily caloric difference between saturated and unsaturated fats has increased over the last 50 years, as researchers claim, these unnecessary calories for men are simply adding more of the wrong kind of fats to their cholesterol levels, in addition to adding surplus weight that increases their risk of high blood pressure.

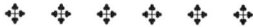

Although the consumption of alcohol contributes to mortality from other causes (for example, accidents and cirrhosis of the liver), it makes only a small contribution to heart disease. In fact, it is now recognized that when consumed at low levels alcohol provides some protection. While most studies show these results with consistency, the reasons that those who have one drink of alcohol per day are at lower risk for heart disease than those who do not drink at all are not clear.

Favourable findings for alcohol are not relevant, however, for those who exceed this moderate level. The National Population Health Survey of 1996-97 defines an excessive amount of alcohol as more than 14 drinks per week for men and more than nine per week for women, and notes that alcohol in excess of these amounts is associated with increased risk of high blood pressure and heart disease.[43] Over eight percent of Canadian men report this level of drinking compared to four percent of Canadian women. The Health

Survey cautions that a tendency for individuals to under-report alcohol consumption may mean that these percentages are slightly lower than reality. To the extent that heart disease takes more lives than any other single cause, however, the fact that twice as many men as women have more than two drinks a day may explain part of their differences in longevity.

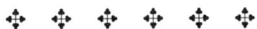

Risk factors have been considered separately here, but there is evidence that many people have more than one risk factor for heart disease. In the 1996-97 health survey two or more risk factors were reported by 41 percent of men and 33 percent of women between 18 and 74 years of age. It is not clear to what extent Canadians are taking steps to reduce those risk factors within their control. Surveyed in 1997, 55 percent of men and 50 percent of women reported they were taking no measures to improve their health.[44] A 1990 U.S. study showed that, while the mortality rate for heart disease had declined over the previous ten years, only 25 percent of the decline was due to controlling risk factors. In contrast, most of the decline (72 percent) was due to early diagnosis, early treatment, and improvements in treatment of the disease once established.[45]

These findings are revealing. They indicate that individuals—and in the case of heart disease that means mostly men—are leaving the substantial part of their cardiovascular health for someone else to worry about. The problem is left to medical researchers and practitioners. There are surely limits to what even that profession can do to clean up the damage we do to ourselves.

CHAPTER 4

Cancer and Lifestyles

Twenty-seven percent of Canadians who die every year die of cancer. Of total cancer deaths in 1997, roughly 61 percent were male and 39 percent female. Male to female ratios are even higher in certain types of cancer, specifically cancers of the lung, esophagus, stomach, and bladder, where there are significant correlations with lifestyles.

There are records of cancer as far back as two thousand years ago, but its place among the leading causes of death is barely a century old. Even before it rose from eighth to second place among causes in developed countries by the mid-twentieth century, many medical practitioners were referring to cancer as a disease of modern civilization. Their observations suggested a strong connection between lifestyles accompanying economic modernization and the rising number of cancer deaths. In particular, frontier doctors and medical missionaries who worked in remote areas of the world reported that they were finding no cases of cancer among primitive people. A quote from Nobel laureate Albert Schweitzer who founded the famous hospital at Lambaréné in Africa is an example:

> On my arrival in Gabon, in 1913, I was astonished to encounter no case of cancer... I can not, of course, say positively that there was no cancer at all, but, like other frontier doctors, I can only say that if any cases existed they must have been quite rare.[46]

As cancer cases in Africa increased in later years, Schweitzer attributed the growing numbers to the fact that "the natives were living more and more after the manner of the whites." Dr. Samuel Hutton, a doctor and missionary among the Labrador eskimos from 1902 to 1913, made similar observations. Returning to practice in Britain following his work in the north, he wrote: "I have not seen or heard of a case of malignant new growth in an Eskimo."[47]

There were also other factors at play. While early frontier doctors attributed the small number of cancer cases to primitive lifestyles, they were practising medicine in a period when most inhabitants of those regions were dying at relatively young ages from infectious diseases and malnutrition. Their observations that cancer could be the result of environmental influences were prophetic, if not entirely based on an accurate comparison of death causes in the two parts of the world. As the century progressed and life expectancies increased the population structure of the world shifted from younger to older. Cancer, predominantly a disease of increasing age, began to take more lives, the majority due to environmental causes in a modern world that even Schweitzer and Hutton could not have predicted.

The rate of cancer incidence rose dramatically from 1900 to the early 1990s and, in the absence of any scientific breakthrough, cancer as a cause of death rose in importance as well. When both rates began to level off and decrease by the 1990s, it was not so much the result of a long-awaited cure as it was the result of discoveries connecting cancer with lifestyles and environmental factors of twentieth century modernization. Among chemical factors, smoking, alcohol consumption, and industrial chemicals are all involved. Non-chemical factors such as sunlight and viral infections are also significant causes of cancer, with increased damage from sunlight especially linked to the influences of modernization on the atmosphere.

These discoveries have pointed to an important role for prevention of disease when cures have not yet been found. Interestingly, while most of the gradual decline in heart disease mortality over the past twenty years has been attributed to earlier medical diagnosis and improvements in treatment, the gradual decline in cancer mortality has been attributed to a large extent to prevention. Changes in lifestyle have shown the most promising results, although cancer still remains the second leading cause of death across the developed world.

In Canada cancer mortality followed the same pattern throughout the twentieth century as it did in other countries. In 1920, the earliest year of record-keeping, most Canadians died of diseases that barely warrant a listing in the mortality tables today. Only 6,800 Canadians died of cancer. In contrast, roughly 13,000 died of influenza, bronchitis and pneumonia; 10,000 of other infectious and parasitic diseases such as diphtheria, whooping cough, typhoid, gastritis, etc.; 10,000 of diseases of early infancy; and 7,700 of tuberculosis.[48] Many of these disease categories have faded into insignificance today. Public health measures aimed at communicable diseases (the use of sera and vaccines) brought the mortality rates from these causes down dramatically in the early part of the century. From the 1920s to the 1940s the mortality rate dropped 100 percent for smallpox, 91 percent for diphtheria, 89 percent for typhoid fever, and 83 percent for childhood diseases like whooping cough, scarlet fever, and measles.[49] In addition, infant mortality was reduced by almost half during the same period as a result of public health improvements.

Mortality rates for cancer, however, continued to rise, partly due to the fact that people were living longer and beginning to die of more degenerative diseases. By the middle of the century approximately 18,000 Canadians died annually of cancer, an increase of 165 percent from 1920, while the Canadian population increased by only 60 percent during the same period. By the 1990s the number of annual deaths from cancer was 65,000.

Even more striking over the years has been the rise in lung cancer in particular. During the 1920s, when cancer of the stomach, liver, and intestines accounted for over 55 percent of all cancer deaths, lung cancer was not even listed.[50] Today it is the leading cause of cancer death among Canadians. In fact, Canada ranks second after the United States in the rate of lung cancer mortality in the world.[51] Lung cancer is also among five types of cancer which take a far greater death toll among men than women. Canadian men are twice as likely to die of lung cancer as women, a ratio that accounts for close to a full year of the six-year gap between their life expectancies, according to epidemiologists. Also contributing to the gap are cancer of the esophagus, stomach, and bladder, all taking the lives of men at more than twice the rate of women, and cancer of the colon at one and a half times the rate. Because of their smaller numbers, the latter four together probably account for another five to six months of the gap.

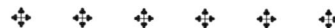

As with heart disease, there are risk factors associated with the development of cancer that are more common to men than to women. Before identifying these risk factors it may be useful to look at what actually happens when a carcinogen or other risk factor initiates the growth and spread of cancer, especially those cancers that end in death.

The development of cancer is essentially an accumulation of damaged or abnormal cells that no longer follow the fairly precise laws of normal cell growth and death. Normal cells carry built-in mechanisms that control their growth, but cancer cells no longer respond to these mechanisms and proliferate beyond control. Normal cells also regulate cell death. Cancer cells can accumulate as a result of the breakdown in this programmed cell death, a breakdown in what has been described as "self-policing mechanisms that activate suicide programs" in normal cells.[52]

The transformation of normal cells with growth and death regulatory mechanisms into cancer cells without regulation is initiated by a carcinogen or a cancer-producing agent. The carcinogenic agents act on the genetic material deoxyribonucleic acid (DNA) of cells, a material that contains the cell's genetic information and is essential for its proper functioning and indeed for the healthy functioning of the whole body. The mechanisms by which these agents act is through direct damage or change, or both, to the DNA—in effect, growth-stimulating genes are continuously switched on and programmed cell death genes are permanently switched off.

It is interesting also that carcinogenic agents may initiate these alterations in the DNA of cells but more than one altered gene is needed for abnormal cells to form a mass, or tumour. In some cases cells that have been transformed initially by a carcinogenic agent may remain latent for a period, and it may take over 20 years in a multi-step process before other genetic changes cause tumours to develop. Completely eliminating exposure to the harmful carcinogen early on can reduce the likelihood of later tumour development.

In the absence of such a reversal, a tumour is eventually formed and begins to grow out of control. Tumour cells originating in a specific organ begin to invade supporting tissues, tissues that carry necessary nutrients to the organ in question. Upon invading these supporting tissues in search of nutrients for their own growth, malignant tumours can travel in the blood or in lymphatic vessels to other parts of the body and develop into secondary tumours in those distant locations. The potential ability of tumour cells to invade surrounding tissues and spread through the vascular and lymphatic systems is what distinguishes malignant from benign tumours.

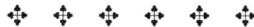

The cancer-producing agents that initiate this deadly process can be physical (for the most part, radiation or ultraviolet light), chemical, or viral. It is now commonly held by experts in the fields of chemistry, environment, epidemiology, and health that 75 to 90 percent of all human cancers are initiated by environmental chemical factors. The predominance of chemical carcinogens explains in part the predominance of men among those who die of cancer. Men are more likely to be exposed to these carcinogens and, in each case, their exposure becomes a major risk factor as the duration and intensity of the exposure increases.

A frequent target of chemical carcinogens is the lung; cancer of the lung today accounts for over a quarter of all cancer deaths in

Canada.[53] This figures is startling when it has been recognized for over 50 years that the major risk factor for lung cancer is tobacco smoking. Both the inhalation of smoke and the chemical content of the tobacco play a role. A healthy lung normally cleans its bronchial tubes by continually moving mucous upward to get rid of any damaging particles inhaled into the body. Smoke inhalation interferes with the mechanisms of this natural process. As a result, damaging substances are not moved on and out; instead they remain trapped in the mucous on the surface lining of the lung.[54] Cancer-producing chemicals in tobacco are among those substances trapped when the lung has lost its cleansing mechanism. Staying too long on the bronchial lining, they eventually pass into the cells beneath where they initiate some form of carcinogen-DNA interaction and subsequent damage that turns formerly normal cells into cancer cells.

This destructive process is happening every day to many Canadian smokers and it happens more frequently to men than to women. Almost 27 percent of Canadian men smoke compared to 23 percent of women.[55] Lung cancer mortality figures show clearly the relationship between smoking and the onset of cancer 20 to 25 years later. In 1975 Quebec had the highest percentage of male smokers (50 percent), today it ranks highest of all provinces in the rate of male lung cancer mortality. The Atlantic provinces had the second highest percentage (45 percent) 25 years ago and today they rank second highest in male lung cancer mortality. The prairie provinces had the lowest percentage (40 percent) and today they rank lowest in male lung cancer mortality, Alberta and Saskatchewan especially having rates well below the Canadian average.

The connection between smoking and lung cancer 20 to 25 years later is also shown in male and female mortality rates during the twentieth century. Male lung cancer mortality began a slow decline in the 1980s, reflecting the fact that male smoking rates reached a peak in the mid-1960s. Female mortality rates from lung cancer, on the other hand, continued to climb while male rates fell, reflecting the peak in female smoking rates in the 1970s.

Cancers in other sites—the bladder, esophagus, throat, and

kidney—also show a strong association with tobacco smoking, the carcinogens in cigarette smoke gaining easy access to the blood stream through the lung. Studies in the United Kingdom, for example, suggest that smoking accounts for about half the cases of bladder cancer, there.[56] A number of aromatic hydrocarbons in cigarette smoke tar are potent carcinogens related to bladder cancer as are many other chemicals identified by medical researchers. Like lung cancer mortality, mortality rates related to these four cancer sites are also twice as high for men as for women.

When we look for chemical causes of cancer, there are other enemies besides smoking. Despite regulations put in place during the late twentieth century, chemical carcinogens inhaled in the course of certain occupations are an important cause of cancer deaths. While industrial sources of cancer do not make as large a contribution to total cancer deaths as smoking, they most certainly affect more men than women and contribute to the predominance of male deaths among lung cancer statistics and among statistics related to other cancer sites.

Statistics, however, are the last thing we think of when we read of human tragedies related to workplace carcinogens. Many Canadian workers exposed to high levels of airborne asbestos fibres during the manufacture of certain building and other products (insulation, fireproofing sheets, wallboard, brake linings, textiles) have died of lung cancer to which they were exposed long before most forms of asbestos were prohibited under federal legislation in 1985 or put under tighter controls. Nonetheless, the long latency period after exposure (from 30 to 40 years) means that asbestos-related lung cancer deaths will continue for years to come.

Workers inhaling high levels of fumes containing aromatic hydrocarbons arising from coke ovens have also died of lung cancer, as have workers exposed to coal tar and coal gas, both by-products of the preparation of coke. (In Canada the first financial compensation for lung cancer deaths among coal gas workers was made in 1949.[57]) Workers have also been exposed to carcinogens in the manufacture or refining of chromates and nickel. Chromium, a known carcinogen, is the source of chromates used as pigments in paints and dyeing and in the tanning of leather. Both chromium and nickel compounds are associated with lung cancer with a latency period averaging 16 years.[58]

Lung cancer is not the only type of cancer affected by industrial chemicals; other cancer sites have been affected. For example, the chemicals used in the dye and rubber industries (proven carcinogens 2-naphthylamine and benzidine, among others) have been shown to cause cancer of the bladder in workers exposed. The chemical, 2-naphthylamine, is particularly carcinogenic.[59] The latency period for this class of chemicals known as the aromatic amines (that is, compounds derived from ammonia) is approximately 15 years on average and can be up to 50 years. Another example is the finding that, in addition to its major target of the respiratory tract, asbestos has caused stomach cancer and colon cancer. And still another type of cancer affected by industrial chemicals is leukemia. Coal tar, mentioned earlier as a by-product in the manufacture of coke, produces the hydrocarbon benzene, commercially used as a solvent, which is one of the two main occupational causes of leukemia (the other is radiation, a physical rather than a chemical carcinogen).[60] Leukemia, a malignancy characterized by an excess of white cells in the blood, can take up to 25 years to develop after exposure.

These were all tragic surprises of modern industry. Even though regulations have been put in place in many cases, the death toll will continue for a while longer. The majority of victims are men (during most of the twentieth century almost all were men), and their deaths contribute to the gap between male and female life expectancies. But the contribution is small; occupational cancers represent from 5 to 10 percent of all cancers.

Whether exposure to occupational hazards can correctly be called lifestyle or behavioural causes of cancer is another question. One cancer researcher found mixed responses to the question of cooperation on the part of workers in complying with protective measures against chemical hazards. In some plants there was no problem. In others, examples of improper use of protective equipment, or total failure to use it, were reported.[61] Given the long latency period for occupational cancer, the compliance question seems academic. Workers continue to be victims of cancer that might have been initiated by industrial sources operating long ago. They were never asked to comply with regulations because, before the dangers were uncovered through medical research, there were no regulations requiring their compliance.

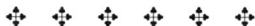

A highly respected study of cancer causes in the 1980s placed alcohol slightly lower than occupational hazards in a list of various factors contributing to cancer. It was estimated that no more than 4 percent of all cancer deaths are attributable to alcohol consumption.[62] This ranking has not been challenged substantially since. There have been many studies, however, showing that the combination of smoking and alcohol consumption is even more deadly than either risk factor alone. This is particularly true in the case of cancers of the esophagus and throat where, in fact, alcohol and smoking combined have been shown to have 12 times the risk for non-smokers and non-drinkers.[63] Moreover, alcohol appears to play the more important role of the two. While smoking alone doubles the risk for esophagal and throat cancer, alcohol alone can have an increased risk seven times greater. Alcohol has also been shown to be a risk factor for cancers of the tongue and mouth and, not surprisingly, it is a risk factor for cirrhosis of the liver which, in turn, is a risk factor for cancer of the liver.

While the carcinogenic damage caused by tobacco and industrial chemicals on human cells (described earlier) has been demonstrated by medical research, the mechanism through which alcohol affects cancer is less well understood. It has been suggested that alcohol facilitates the development of cancer by increasing the contact between these carcinogens and cells of the esophagus, throat, and mouth, etc.[64] It has also been suggested that alcohol may suppress the immune system; alternatively, or even at the same time, may contribute to malnutrition which could make the alcohol consumer more vulnerable to malignant change. Whatever the mechanisms, statistics of alcohol use and cancer mortality suggest that moderate amounts of alcohol consumption are not a cancer risk.

For all these major cancer sites associated with excess alcohol consumption—esophagus, throat, liver, tongue, and mouth—the mortality rates for men are considerably higher than for women, as much as four and a half times higher in the case of throat cancer.[65] When these statistics are compared to statistics on alcohol consumption among Canadians, they are easier to understand. Over eight percent of Canadian men report having more than 14 drinks per week compared to four percent of women.[66] In addition, well over half of men who drink report having five or more drinks on any one occasion compared to one-third of women. Men might drink this heavily 19 times during a year, on average, while women do so an average of eight times.[67]

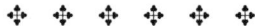

Diet as a risk factor for cancer has been suggested many times by comparing the incidence of cancer in various countries, a commonly used method of present-day epidemiologists (and less scientifically by early frontier doctors comparing primitive and non-primitive people a hundred years ago). For example, in Japan the incidence of colon cancer is much lower than in the U.S., including Hawaii; yet studies of Japanese who have moved to Hawaii have found an increased fat intake and a much increased risk of colon cancer. This and other examples point to a strong correlation between per capita fat consumption and cancer of the colon. Although such population comparisons are suggestive, they require additional corroboration from longitudinal studies of specific individuals before they are conclusive, and such studies are extremely difficult. Individual diet histories are usually the source of information on dietary intakes over long periods, a methodology plagued with inaccuracies.

Despite these difficulties, as early as 1982 the National Academy of Sciences in the U.S. concluded that of all the dietary components studied by scientists, the evidence was most strongly in support of fat intake as a cancer risk factor.[68] The Academy also considered the possible contribution of low fibre intake. Although there were individual studies linking high-fibre diets with low risk of colon cancer, results were inconsistent and fell short of providing conclusive evidence that fibre protects against colon cancer. Over the next 20 years experimental studies continued, and today it has been acknowledged, following the most recent research, that fibre has little effect on reducing colon cancer risk.

As with cancer-producing agents from other sources, carcinogens in the human diet initiate cancer by damaging DNA. It is believed dietary carcinogens generate free oxygen radicals, which in turn may be responsible for the damage.[69] This oxidizing damage has given rise to an important field of cancer research, the search for mechanisms (also in the human diet) which protect body cells from oxidation—mechanisms known as anti-oxidants. Vitamin E and beta-carotene are known anti-oxidants; tea has also been shown to be rich in anti-oxidants. Studies have also demonstrated that dietary lycopene in tomatoes, especially when they are processed into juices and other products, has anti-oxidant properties.[70]

These various findings implicate diet as a source of cancer-producing agents as well as of protective mechanisms. But if there is a typical Canadian diet—indeed a typical North American diet—why do these carcinogens affect only some of us? Men in Canada are twice as likely as women to die of stomach cancer and more than one and a half times as likely to die of colon cancer, both cancer sites that are clearly major parts of the digestive system affected by diet.[71] And there are further unexplained discrepancies. Canadian statistics show gradual declines in both stomach and colon cancer over the last 30 years, which may be due to changes in dietary habits of the general population. Still, male-female differences persist in one of these declines. While stomach cancer has decreased at equal rates for both men and women, colon cancer has decreased by 43 percent for Canadian women during that period but by only 20 percent for men.[72]

A partial explanation for these differences may be a greater tendency for men to be overweight, especially when excess weight is considered a risk factor for some types of cancer. In 1999 roughly

42 percent of Canadian men were overweight, measured by body mass index,[73] compared to 24 percent of women.[74] Clearly many men are taking in more calories than they need, and it is probable that some part of the excess weight is a result of taking in a disproportionate share of dietary fat. Although the contribution of dietary factors as a cause of cancer is still being explored, the association of fat intake and excess weight with cancer could be another piece of the puzzle of shorter lifespans for men.

One can also look to genetic factors in trying to explain why carcinogens affect only some of us. At the basis of a genetic explanation, hereditary deficiencies can result in differential handling of toxins. In addition, a series of accumulating genetic changes in cells takes place in cancer progression, some genetic changes causing uncontrolled cell growth or inhibition of cell death, and others causing tumour invasion and spread. Whether there is a difference in the way these changes are played out in men and women is still unknown.

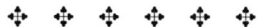

Bringing world nations together in 1997 to discuss health and mortality, the United Nations identified stages, or transitions, of significant mortality decline over the past century.[75] The first transition involved the decline in mortality from infectious diseases in developed countries in the early 1900s as a result of the vaccines and public health measures mentioned earlier. The second transition came with the decline in mortality due to cardiovascular disease since the 1970s. (In Canada the mortality rate for cardiovascular disease today is half what it was in 1970.) While much of this progress is due to improvements in medical diagnosis and treatment, the UN acknowledged that this transition also confirms the importance of behavioural changes in achieving mortality reductions. The next transition, according to the UN, is yet to occur. It involves the reduction in cancer as a cause of death—indeed in several developed countries cancer rates are already dropping. With its high male to female ratio, the decline of cardiovascular disease mortality has already started to narrow the gap between male and female longevity, and cancer declines are expected to make it even narrower, at least in the short term. These developments will come at later stages in less advanced countries where the first transition, the decline in mortality from infectious diseases, occurred only in the last decades of the twentieth century.

Chapter 5

Lung and Liver Diseases and Lifestyles

No matter how one arranges the figures to assess the damage, smoking and heavy drinking come out on top as major contributors to the gap between male and female life expectancies. This has become true in many countries of the world, even though the progression toward longer lifespans in general is uneven due to wide variations in economic development and the resources to achieve it.

Although heart disease is now the leading cause of death across the developed world, the death toll from infectious diseases has not been overcome in many developing regions, as it has in advanced regions after 40 or 50 years of antibiotics and other controls. By 1990 roughly 42 percent of deaths in the developing world were caused by infectious diseases, compared to only six percent in the advanced regions.[76] Even as mortality from infectious diseases starts to come down, however, developing countries have already started to experience the negative fallout of modernization, including the increasing importance of so-called lifestyle diseases for which antibiotics are not the answer. And the worst is yet to come. Smoking has reached such proportions in developing countries that World Health Organization (WHO) researchers now call it the "tobacco epidemic." The WHO estimates that in 1990 alone the world death toll from smoking was three million people, with the majority of deaths still in the developed world. However, the recent rapid increase in tobacco use in Asia and other developing regions is expected to kill many more people in the coming decades than have so far died in the developed regions.[77]

The situation with alcohol is not so straightforward. It has been shown to provide some protection against heart disease but to increase the risk of other diseases and to cause many accidental deaths. Because of its protective effect against heart disease, alcohol probably prevents about as many deaths as it causes in advanced countries. In many developing countries the picture is different: with lower death rates from heart disease, alcohol caused over 600,000 more deaths than it prevented in developing countries in 1990, the year of the WHO study.

And the bad news is not entirely in for the developed world. Although the most visible outcome from smoking during the twentieth century was the increase in lung cancer, the connection between smoking and heart disease covered in an earlier chapter actually accounted for most smoking-related deaths because of the sheer number of heart disease deaths throughout the world. In addition, there has been a slow steady growth in mortality from other diseases linked to smoking, most notably respiratory diseases. As an editorial in the medical journal *Lancet* points out, cancer of the lung is not the whole story. For every tobacco-associated death from lung cancer there are two or three from other diseases.[78] These diseases and deaths affect men three times more frequently than they affect women—an estimated 1.5 million tobacco-associated deaths for men in developed countries in 1995, compared to half a million for women. Besides the toll taken by tobacco as a risk factor for these diseases, alcohol use in excess continues to be a risk factor for liver cirrhosis, with men twice as likely as women to drink heavily and twice as likely to die of liver cirrhosis. Consequently the gains in lifespans in developed countries after more than a century of modernization are not as large as they could be, and once again it is men who fail to make the gains.

As in other developed countries, heart disease and cancer have been leading causes of death in Canada for several decades. Tobacco and heavy alcohol use have long since been identified as risk factors. Significantly, these two diseases and these two risk factors are more common to Canadian men than to women; together they account for a good portion of the six-year gap in male-female life expectancies. Some researchers have estimated as high a portion as two to three years. Canada also lists respiratory disease and liver cirrhosis among its leading causes of death, as do other developed countries. These diseases kill many more men than women and account for an additional portion of the life expectancy gap, perhaps as much as six to eight months. With respiratory disease consistently linked to smoking (American studies have shown that smokers are six times more likely to develop bronchitis and emphysema than non-smokers) and liver cirrhosis consistently linked to alcohol abuse, the lethal consequences of these two lifestyles for Canadians continue to be a depressing reality.

A closer look at trends in mortality rates and mortality causes related to respiratory disease and liver cirrhosis completes the picture of the major life style diseases that rose to importance in the twentieth century.

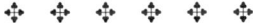

To describe respiratory diseases briefly it is simpler to divide them into chronic and acute diseases, since the various chronic categories are most often directly attributed to smoking. At the same time, acute respiratory diseases—especially pneumonia—may be indirectly linked to smoking by virtue of the fact that those with chronic lung disease are prime candidates for such infections. Nonetheless, chronic respiratory diseases (or chronic obstructive pulmonary diseases) are those at the forefront in any discussion of smoking.

Chronic respiratory diseases cover a range of lung diseases, some identified by name in Canadian mortality statistics and most simply identified as "chronic airways obstruction." All are characterized by difficult breathing or some other indication that the body's respiratory system has become out of tune. When operating properly the respiratory system, including the lungs, brings in air containing oxygen that is carried from the lungs through the bloodstream to be used as fuel by cells in all parts of the body. The cells, in turn, give off carbon dioxide, which is carried back to the lungs to be eliminated or exhaled.

This vital process accomplished by the lungs has built-in defense responses to infection or to irritants that may disrupt the system.[79] In the normal course of events, the respiratory system's defenses will protect against inhaled harmful substances such as dirt or germs—coughing, sneezing or filtering them, moving them out of the lungs in mucous, or putting special scavenger cells to work that literally eat them up. When things go wrong in this intricate process, the lungs cannot do their work properly.

The major cause of chronic problems in the respiratory system is cigarette smoking. People who smoke are those most likely to develop bronchitis, for example, an inflammation of the lining of the bronchial tubes that connect the windpipe with the lungs. For a start, smoke irritates the bronchial tubes and over a long period of time causes the production of excessive mucous, thickening of the tube linings, and a persistent cough. In the meantime, gases and particles in the inhaled smoke have slowed down the workings of tiny, microscopic hairs in the bronchial tubes whose function is to move dirt and germs out of the lungs. When this happens as a result of long-term smoking, the ability of the lungs to defend themselves against infection is weakened.

Another well-known example of respiratory disease is emphysema, a condition related to the tiny air sacs at the end of the bronchial tubes where oxygen is transferred to the bloodstream. Smoking upsets an important balance between chemicals in the lungs, destroying in the process the elastic fibres that allow the lungs to expand and contract and creating permanent holes in the fragile air sacs. As the damage continues, the lungs are able to transfer less and less oxygen to the bloodstream, causing the shortness of breath that is characteristic of emphysema.

Inhaled smoke also closes up air passages, making breathing more difficult and clearly worsening the situation for those with bronchial asthma, a condition of chronic inflammation in the lungs that causes the bronchial tubes and their branches to constrict from time to time. The tightness in the chest and breathing difficulty associated with asthma may be triggered by any number of allergens, but the ability of smoking to inflame the lungs' airways on its own aggravates the problem.

Although smoking is the major cause of these malfunctions, other factors can also disrupt the respiratory system. Asthma can be triggered by cold weather, allergies, overexertion, and sometimes workplace chemicals. Inherited factors can also play a role. Both chronic bronchitis and emphysema can be caused by irritants over a long period of time such as air pollution and industrial fumes and dusts. All of these causes, however, are secondary in importance to smoking.

In contrast to chronic forms, acute respiratory diseases, especially bacterial pneumonia, can often be treated with antibiotics (which are not effective with viral pneumonias). The antibiotics can control bacteria that have worked their way into the lungs and inflamed the air sacs, filling the lungs or part of the lungs with liquid matter. Besides antibiotics, vaccines are also available. These medical advances have been responsible for the decline in pneumonia deaths in Canada and all developed countries in the last half of the twentieth century. Despite these declines, pneumonia is not expected to drop out of sight in developed countries over the next decade, where it will be ranked in importance only slightly lower than chronic respiratory diseases. While declines were being recorded in the developed world, pneumonia remained the leading cause of death in the developing world up to the end of the century. Declines in those regions are expected over the next ten years.

In Canada chronic respiratory disease ranks third in causes of death after cardiovascular disease and cancer. Over the past 20 years trends in mortality from respiratory disease have followed trends in smoking two decades earlier, in a similar pattern to that of lung cancer mortality. Male mortality from respiratory disease rose steadily until the late 1980s when it began to decline following the peak and decline in male smoking rates in the mid-1960s. Female smoking rates peaked a decade later, with the result that female mortality from respiratory disease continued to rise in the late 1980s and has only recently started to level off.

Health Canada has completed biennial studies of mortality

attributed to tobacco use in Canada since 1988. The latest study shows that a total of 45,000 deaths in 1996 can be attributed to smoking, or one-fifth of all deaths that year. An equal share of tobacco-related deaths can be attributed to each of cardiovascular disease and cancer (39 percent each), 16 percent to chronic respiratory disease and another five percent to pneumonia and influenza.[80] Smoking that led to chronic respiratory diseases accounted for over 7,200 deaths in Canada in 1996. Of those deaths, roughly 4,500 were male and 2,700 female, or one and two-thirds times more male than female tobacco-related deaths from chronic respiratory disease. While this disadvantage for men may give cause for concern, the ratio has come down from three to one in the 1960s and 1970s, with the earlier decline in male smoking rates.

In the meantime, according to Health Canada, smoking remains the number one preventable cause of death and disease in Canada, far exceeding by five times the second most preventable cause of death—accidents. The Health Canada estimates of 45,000 smoking-related deaths across the country in 1996 are almost identical to earlier predictions for Canada made by the World Health Organization. WHO also predicted that smoking-related deaths will continue to rise worldwide over the next 20 years. Chronic respiratory disease, among other implicated diseases, will double by 2020 largely due to the impact of tobacco use in developing countries.

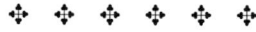

Modern lifestyles have affected the human lung over the last century and have taken many lives prematurely in the process. Another vital part of the body that can be fatally damaged by lifestyle choices is the liver. In the case of the liver, however, alcohol rather than tobacco is the culprit.

The liver lacks some of the glamour of the heart and lungs, its description often becoming bogged down in detail because of the complicated role it plays in the body. One academic has suggested that one of the basic texts on the liver has all the intellectual excitement of an army manual on weaponry.[81] A very brief account, therefore, of the liver's role in the body will serve to demonstrate the connection between liver cirrhosis and alcohol.

The functions of the liver are numerous—it stores and filters blood, forms and secretes bile, excretes pigments left over from old red blood cells, and converts proteins and fats into glucose, among many other essential functions. The liver performs all these functions by receiving blood from the heart through one route and from the stomach and intestines through another, performing its multi-faceted work, and then passing the blood on through to the heart. Needless to say, a liver failing to carry out all these tasks properly will interfere with the basic functioning of the whole body and can lead to death.

The complicated workings of the liver take place in an organ weighing between three and four pounds and made up of a maze of interconnected cell walls, canals, veins, capillaries, and bile ducts. When the liver's shape and the maze of inner connections, appropriately called its architecture by medical scientists, are disturbed or distorted, the flow of blood through the liver can back up or be blocked. Cirrhosis, the liver disease capable of inflicting this kind of damage on the liver's architecture, has a long latency period and is normally irreversible.

The important role of alcohol in the development of cirrhosis is not surprising, given that the liver is where most drugs and toxins, including alcohol, are metabolized. In the process, and especially when an excess of alcohol is taken in, liver cells can be damaged or destroyed. The dead cells regenerate, forming small nodules separated by membranes of connective tissue which cause permanent scarring. The membranes also act as impenetrable barriers, obstructing blood vessels and causing the breakdown of the liver's many functions.

Alcohol abuse is the most common cause of liver cirrhosis in the U.S., Canada, Australia, and western Europe. Chronic hepatitis can also be a cause; in fact, hepatitis B is the principal cause of liver cirrhosis in Africa and many parts of Asia. Nutritional deficiencies are not blamed as frequently as they used to be but may still be a cause of cirrhosis in some cases. For these reasons the World Health

Organization has made a mixed bag of predictions about liver cirrhosis over the next 20 years. It is expected to increase in developed countries where alcohol is a popular lifestyle choice and, of course, where more affluence allows such choices to be made. It is expected to decrease in India, China, Africa, and the middle East.[82] These scenarios suggest a certain amount of optimism about lower rates of hepatitis B and better nutrition throughout the world and a continuing pessimism about alcohol abuse.

In Canada liver cirrhosis ranks fifth in causes of death after cardiovascular disease, cancer, respiratory diseases, and accidents. Mortality from cirrhosis has declined slightly over the past 30 years, with much of the decline attributed to lower rates for men. During that time Canadian men have been more than twice as likely as women to die of liver cirrhosis. This ratio continues today. Similarly their rates of alcohol consumption have been higher; in 1995 over 58 percent of men who drank were heavy drinkers compared to 33 percent of women.[83] Considering that alcohol in moderation is now recognized as a preventive for heart disease, alcohol in excess wipes out the gains, especially for men, and makes a considerable contribution to keeping them in second place in life expectancy comparisons.

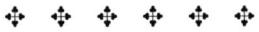

Health researchers use a simple method to determine the impact of tobacco on mortality. They estimate the total number of deaths that would have occurred in a given year if everyone had died at the same rate as non-smokers. This hypothetical figure is then compared with the number of deaths that actually occurred. The excess deaths can, without too much argument, be attributed to smoking. Fewer such comparisons have been made about the impact of alcohol. Information about alcohol use may be less reliable, especially when the information needed is alcohol abuse rather than alcohol use. (As mentioned earlier, it now appears that alcohol in moderation can be beneficial to health, whereas there have been no comparable claims for the virtues of moderate smoking.) In addition, the primary "alcohol abuse" disease is liver cirrhosis, accounting for fewer deaths than heart disease, cancer, and respiratory disease and possibly yielding less dramatic impact figures than those related to tobacco. Despite the need for more alcohol-related studies, the available national and international impact studies show the importance of lifestyle causes to mortality rates, and consistently show that the excess deaths from such causes are largely male.

From the male perspective, it is not enough that they are dying earlier; they are also blamed for their bad luck. This seems a fair observation. And yet in all the articles giving cold statistics of the disproportionate share of self-destructive lifestyles among men (most articles written by top-notch male medical researchers) the reasons for choosing such lifestyles are rarely covered. Admittedly, research is increasingly zeroing in on tobacco and alcohol—especially tobacco—as the strongest risk factors for mortality worldwide. The findings are also presented more confidently than in the past, allowing no room for alternative interpretation. Still there seems to be a reluctance to dig deeper to find motives. It is hardly enough to conclude that the better economic position of men across the world allows them to indulge in expensive lifestyles. Or that it is more socially acceptable for them to do so.

In the absence of convincing motives, there are some clues in the research literature on addiction. The addictive qualities of tobacco and alcohol help to explain their prevalence in developed countries for almost a century and their growing importance in developing countries today, despite the vast amount of public information about their consequences. Where the use of tobacco or alcohol is no longer under an individual's voluntary control, it qualifies as addiction. Considering the medical and social harm that can be caused, one medical researcher has called addiction a disorder of motivation.[84]

But are men more inclined either biologically or psychologically toward addictive behaviour than women? U.S. studies examining addictions have found sex differences at the early stage of involvement in drug use, with males more likely than females to have an opportunity to use drugs in the first place. Females, however, are just as likely as males to make the transition into regular drug use once the initial opportunity has occurred. In other words, greater male involvement in drug use and addiction could be accounted for by greater male exposure to initial drug opportunities. A similar explanation might apply to tobacco and alcohol addictions.

An increasing number of addiction researchers have also found evidence to suggest that some individuals may be genetically vulnerable to addictive behaviour. A "dopamine receptor" gene is suspected.[85] The idea of genetic markers for "novelty-seeking" behaviour that predispose people to take chances is relatively recent and might be added to the equation some day. There is no suggestion so far that this gene is found more often in males than in females.

In the meantime, long before these advances in genetic research, considerable research has taken place on the subject of risk-taking not necessarily associated with addiction. General findings have been that men are greater risk-takers than women. This tendency may be at the root of lifestyle choices that lead to higher death rates for certain diseases, and it has long been acknowledged to be at the root of higher death rates for accidents, to be covered in more detail in the following chapter.

CHAPTER 6

The Risk-takers

A review of the vast medical research into the leading causes of death—and more specifically, into the risk factors linked to each cause of death—is not complete without a consideration of risk-taking itself. It is true that knowledge of risk factors is an important part of disease prevention. It has been shown over the past three decades that health information has influenced the behaviour of many Canadians, and indeed many people in other advanced countries. They have taken steps to cut back on risk factors such as smoking, alcohol, obesity, etc., in the interests of longer life once they became convinced that smoking, alcohol, and obesity could make life shorter.

But knowledge is not the entire solution. Even when the risks are known, many still hang on to these potentially harmful behaviours simply because risks are *risks*. There may be a high probability that they will occur, but there is less than 100 percent certainty. That gap of uncertainty and the rewards of keeping favourite lifestyles (there could even be a happy ending without giving them up) lure the risk-takers. Moreover, the rewards appear within reach, not at some distant point in the future by which time a whole range of events could have intervened, including death from an entirely unrelated cause. Studies of how we perceive time when making such decisions have shown that our perceptions are far from rational; time intervals close to the present seem larger than those in both the past and the future. Given these time distortions, there is a strong argument that the most distant practical horizon for most people is 10 to 15 years.[86]

Not only do time intervals close to the present appear larger, the potential rewards in that time space are more valued even though larger rewards could be achieved in the longer term. A comment often attributed to Mark Twain is an example of the magnitude of immediate rewards. When told he could add five years to his life if he gave up smoking and drinking, Twain replied that five years without smoking and drinking were not worth living.[87]

Risk-taking is a human trait of great interest to the insurance industry, health care professionals, investors, personnel recruiters, hazard control agencies, highway traffic engineers, and a host of others. Although an important concern in all these fields, however, it continues to frustrate the efforts of the experts trying to manage it. There is a grudging consensus that, even when supplied with all the statistical help available in the world, individuals view the risk in any given situation from their own personal perspective. In the health field, for example, rational decision-making is often clouded by an unrealistic optimism about personal risk, a tendency for people to underestimate their own health risks compared to the risks of others.[88]

Called "optimism bias" by those studying risk, unrealistic optimism may be a general human tendency, but clearly its strength varies from individual to individual. Figures on the probability of a particular health threat may be available, but people will make decisions about the risk to themselves based on their own perceptions of how susceptible they are to the health threat, how severe the threat is, and whether preventive action is likely to change things.[89] In other words, the weighing of dangers and benefits is not done objectively (or identically) by each individual decision-maker. Instead people see the world quite differently based on their own past experiences and, as a result, their behaviours in the face of risk will be just as varied.

Individual differences in risk-taking are also complicated by the fact that there are tendencies for age and sex to play a role. The past experience of older people might have the effect of emphasizing the dangers and de-emphasizing the benefits of risks. On the other hand, the past experience of younger people may not be as varied, leaving them vulnerable to poor estimates of the magnitude of risks or the importance of the consequences. For some or all of these reasons, the rate of risk-taking tends to decrease as people age.

In the same way, to the extent that male and female roles in society provide different experiences for each gender, they also provide different views of risk-taking. This connection with experience suggests that traits like risk-taking may be learned. Psychologists no longer argue, as they did 50 years ago, that there are innate biologically-based personality traits distinctive to men and women. If any innate differences have held up through numerous experimental studies they are that males are more aggressive than females and that a group of personality traits adding up to action and achievement are more likely to be associated with men while a group of traits adding up to warmth and sensitivity are more likely to be associated with females.[90]

The more important finding over the years of psychological research has been that the behaviours of boys and girls and men and women are strongly influenced by their environment, more specifically by sex stereotypes learned during early socialization in the family and at school. Socializing agents (parents, teachers, etc.) pass on their own perceptions of typical male and female behaviours. It has been found that as early as five years of age children have learned to differentiate between male and female sex roles, activities and characteristics. And despite the millions of parents and teachers perpetuating their own views, there is a remarkable similarity in the stereotypes handed down in any given society, suggesting that they are firmly embedded in the culture of that society.[91] Moreover, adults have very clear expectations about the characteristics of young boys versus girls and these undisguised expectations can channel the behaviour of these young learners in ways that finally confirm the stereotypes. In other words, expectations can be self-fulfilling in their effects on those being socialized.[92] This different socialization for boys and girls is widespread cross-culturally, explaining much of the gender differences in behaviour not only here but in other countries of the world.

The idea of a learned set of beliefs about typical behaviours is useful in understanding why a behaviour like risk-taking should have a stronger tendency to show up in males than in females. The male stereotype of aggression, violence and daring is a key component of the beliefs held by most North Americans about men's behaviour.[93] And not surprisingly, men confirm these beliefs again and again by taking greater risks. Their predominance in taking risks that are clearly linked to the leading fatal diseases has been shown in previous chapters. They are more likely to smoke, drink, overeat, and hold hazardous jobs than are women. There is even stronger evidence of their role as risk-takers in accident statistics, not only in North America but world-wide. These statistics warrant some attention if only because accidents are among the five leading causes of death in most countries of the world.

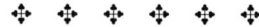

An indication of the extent to which male risk-taking has become part of the culture of Western as well as of many non-Western societies is the dramatic difference in male and female death rates as a result of accidents. According to United Nations data, death rates for accidents and other violent causes have been higher for males than for females in almost all available historical and international data. Ratios of male to female accident mortality have been as high as four to one in Chile, for example, and as low as 1.2 to one in Guatemala, but always greater than one. In the U.S. male-female ratios in the 1990s were still over two to one, as they were 60 years ago. Across the world and across time higher male-female ratios have held for every age group from childhood to old age, with ratios well over three to one for accident victims between the ages of 15 and 45 years.[94]

In Canada the ratios have been just as dramatic as in other countries. In every age group male accidental death rates are greater than female rates. When they first peak in the early 20s, male rates are four and a third times those of women and continue to be four times as high until age 40.[95] Because accidents are the leading cause of death for Canadians under 40, this ratio has a significant impact on differences in life expectancy.

Young people are not the only ones who die accidentally. Accidental death rates peak again after age 65, following a decline in middle age, and the pattern of higher rates for men continues, older men having twice the likelihood as women of dying from accidents. The accident peak in older years, however, is overshadowed by the higher death rates among the elderly for degenerative diseases such as heart disease and cancer. In fact, accidental deaths are only two percent of deaths among the elderly, compared with 75 percent of deaths among those in their late teens and early 20s.[96]

Accidents without fatal consequences are just as revealing of male risk-taking as those ending in death. Generally, men have higher rates than women.[97] Breaking down non-fatal accidents by category shows similar higher rates for men in motor vehicle (one and a half times higher), sports (twice as high), and work accidents (two and a half times as high), although women have higher rates for accidents occurring in the home.

While non-fatal accidents allow statisticians to estimate activity-loss days and even bed-disability days for the whole of Canada, fatal accidents provide statistics in potential years of life lost and the impact on life expectancy. Looking further into why men are losing more potential years of life than women as a result of accidents, the fact that 36 percent of all accident fatalities in Canada are motor vehicle fatalities provides a good portion of the answer.[98] Ever since the automobile became Canada's most popular mode of transportation early in the twentieth century, it has become painfully clear that the speed and convenience it provided came at a huge price in human lives. Automobile driving, like war, is an activity involving high risks. Over 42,000 Canadians died during World War II; an even greater number died on Canada's roads throughout the 1970s when traffic fatalities reached their peak.

Despite a rather formidable accumulation of traffic fatality statistics over the past century, men have not appeared to adjust their level of vigilance to the same extent that women have. With equal access to the same accident statistics, they are inclined to give more weight to speed and convenience than to the potential dangers and more inclined to overestimate their own skill and judgment in the face of a dangerous situation on the road than women do. The result has been consistently higher motor vehicle fatality rates for men over the years. Even as women became more frequent drivers following World War II, men continued to pile up fatality rates in traffic accidents that were almost three times the rates of women (and over four times among young people). There is little evidence that men have failed to note the fatality data; they have simply been more willing to take risks.

Closely related to risk-taking, and its basis in decision-making that is not always rational, is the tragic connection between drinking and driving. In the 1990s Statistics Canada reported that in just one year 1,600 Canadians lost their lives in alcohol-related motor vehicle accidents. Among drivers killed on roads across the country over half had been drinking.[99] A majority of male fatally injured drivers (53 percent) had been drinking compared to 27 percent of females. These figures are even more significant when added to the finding that in one year there were 700 fatally injured drinking drivers who were men, over eight times the number (84) who were women.[100] Men, therefore, made up 90 percent of fatally injured drinking drivers. Other studies showed that men represented 90 to 95 percent of drivers arrested for drinking and driving offenses which did not result in driver fatalities. Not surprisingly, a fact behind these figures is that men make up 80 percent of night-time drivers, a high risk group for alcohol-related accidents.

As the twentieth century ended, traffic fatalities began to drop. Rather impressive figures on decreased mortality—even as the number of drivers and the number of registered automobiles increased—showed annual deaths on Canadian roads dropped from 6,700 in the early 1970s to roughly 3,000 by 1999, a 35-year low. This decrease of well over 50 percent (even higher for men than for women) has been attributed to many factors: lower speed limits, increased use of seat belts, and improvements to automobile and roadway design. But a considerable portion of the decrease in the number of motor vehicle fatalities has to be attributed to a reduction in the number of impaired drivers. For every 100,000 Canadians, the number charged with impaired driving in 1993, for example, was 322 compared to 588 per 100,000 charged in 1978.[101]

An important contribution to the decline in impaired driving has been the trend toward more moderate drinking among Canadians in general. Small declines in heavy drinking occurred between the 1980s and the 1990s (from 51 percent of all drinkers to 46 percent) and the proportion of Canadians who drink at all has dropped from 84 percent to 74 percent. In addition, the average number of drinks consumed per drinker is down, though only slightly, from five drinks a week to four.[102] Sales data across the country also show declining per capita consumption since 1980. These trends explain some of the decrease in automobile fatalities. And figures related to male drinking, in particular, have even more relevance. While the proportion of women drinkers has declined to a greater extent than the proportion of men over the period, men have shown a larger drop in the number of drinks consumed per week. Admittedly they had further to drop, but such figures may be indicative of a trend.

As alcohol use has decreased gradually, the use of seat belts may also have been affected. Past surveys have shown that men, and drinking drivers in particular, are less likely than other drivers to comply with seat belt laws. These survey findings are not surprising. As long as seat belts have to be personally buckled by the car occupant, driver attitudes toward risk come into play.[103] It is possible that reduced alcohol consumption may not only reduce risk-taking on the road based on impaired judgment, but may change driver attitudes toward seat belts before starting out.

The decline in motor vehicle fatalities has been the primary reason for a decline in total accidental deaths in Canada over the past 20 years. Accidental falls are the second major cause of accident mortality, and mortality rates due to falls have changed only slightly over the period, with gains by men offset by higher rates for women. Rates for poisoning deaths are up somewhat and rates for drowning and suffocation down; for both these causes of accidental death, men's rates are twice as high as women's. Changes in rates, however, have tended to cancel each other out. As a result, any net contribution from causes other than traffic fatalities to narrowing the gap between male and female life expectancies has been negligible.

Although suicide is included in accidents in Canadian mortality statistics, it has been excluded in all of the above comparisons because suicide, by definition, is intentional. It is less a decision involving risk and uncertainty than a decision with certain and very final results. Nonetheless, suicide is associated with risk-taking behaviour in its self-destructive aspects, and the same predominance of males exists. Canadian male suicide rates are four times female rates.[104] Men make up almost 80 percent of all suicides in Canada. They have maintained that proportion for over 50 years as suicide rates have climbed, making the finding of a federal government task force that "suicides do not form, as may be thought, a wholly distinct group" somewhat puzzling.[105] Moreover, the task force identifies "high risk" groups for suicide as those with mental disorders, alcoholics, certain age groups, native peoples, persons in custody, and the bereaved, failing to mention men of all ages, men among those suffering from mental disorders, and men of all ethnic, incarcerated and grieving groups.

In 1990 the World Health Organization estimated that worldwide about five million people died of injuries of all types (including suicide), two-thirds of them men. Road traffic accidents and self-inflicted injuries were among the ten leading causes of death in developed regions of the world; road traffic accidents had also broken into the list of top ten causes of death in developing regions. In the world as a whole, because of dramatic increases in accidental deaths in developing countries, road traffic accidents took as many lives as lung cancer. Both, however, still caused only one-sixth of the number of deaths caused by heart disease.[106]

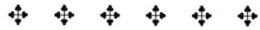

Risk-taking and the predominance of men among risk-takers are highly visible in accidental deaths. Yet less visibly and sometimes over a longer period, risk-taking also plays an important part in premature death from disease. It provides the common thread running through the major leading causes of death—heart disease, cancer, respiratory diseases, liver cirrhosis, and accidents—and because of its fatal consequences, risk takers are often seen as irrational and irresponsible.[107]

In a recent book, simply called *Risk*, John Adams puts risk-taking in a more generous light. Since men are more likely to take risks than women, it is an interesting approach to male behaviour that would otherwise be seen as perverse and self-destructive. Adams argues that a propensity to take risks exists in all of us. Everyone willingly takes risks to satisfy a universal need for a certain amount of excitement in our lives. Too much certainty, according to Adams, is "boring, unrewarding, and belittling."[108] Nonetheless, if uncertainty helps us escape boredom there are some who like it more than others. What distinguishes risk-takers may be a greater concern for keeping their own personalities intact or, more specifically, for holding fast to their personal beliefs. Rather than being irresponsible, risk-taking behaviour may reflect a philosophy that our personal destinies are within our control. The opposing philosophy that some pre-arranged master plan is in place for each of us would be a red flag taunting the risk-taker. Predestination, with its argument that we are all powerless in the hands of fate, rules out the crucial freedom of making choices.

The risk-takers are, in effect, confirming their right to independent choice in their lives, their right to be responsible for their own actions, even their right to be irrational whether their behaviour brings injury to themselves or not. For many people, this may be carrying freedom of choice too far. Without this freedom to do battle with fate, however, it could be argued that powerlessness—uncomfortably close to impotence in the minds of men—can chip away at the precious commodity of personality and individuality. Perhaps male risk-takers treasure their individuality more than the rest of us do.

Chapter 7

Mortality by Marital Status and Social Class

Explaining why men die earlier than women by exploring the roles and lifestyles of human society has brought medical and social sciences closer together. Research has involved biologists, demographers, epidemiologists, geneticists, gerontologists, psychologists, and sociologists. There are compelling pieces of evidence pointing to an interdependence between long life and social factors that have been brought to light in many of these studies. The connection between mortality and marital status and the connection between mortality and social class are the two with the most conclusive findings while others are increasingly receiving the attention of researchers.

The connection between mortality and marital status has now been well established. Despite all the stresses in a social institution that is increasingly breaking down, it appears that marriage is keeping many people alive. Studies in the U.S., U.K., Canada, Sweden, and Finland have shown that unmarried individuals have higher death rates than married individuals. Some of these studies have used vital statistics from government sources; some have been longitudinal studies following cohorts of individuals over one or two decades. Whatever the data source, findings suggest that the social support given by one marriage partner to another provides some protection against death. And the reverse—the unmarried may be inclined toward negative health behaviours in the absence of such social supports.

New studies have followed to test these assumptions with remarkable similarity in their findings. The major Canadian study by gerontologists John Hirdes and William Forbes in 1992 looked at the social supports provided in marriage and added others to test the combined effect of several social relationships on mortality. They created a "social relationships" index made up of marital status, number of living children, weekly contact with family and relatives, and participation in voluntary associations. Results of the study showed a significant association between the social relationships index and mortality, with subjects scoring lowest on the index having the greatest risk of death.

Why social relationships should contribute to health and longevity requires more than one answer. Primarily, social supports are considered important in coping with stressful life events to which we are all exposed from time to time and which, in a general way, can contribute to illness. More specifically, stress has been linked to negative effects on the immune system, even the gastrointestinal system[109] and, as we have seen in an earlier chapter, on the cardiovascular system. In most social relationships, the support given by one individual to another can provide a buffer against these impacts and other damage left in the wake of stressful events.

The argument is also made that social relationships—family and marriage relationships in particular—involve a sense of obligation that inhibits negative health behaviours and promotes positive ones.[110] In other words, the presence of a spouse discourages activities that could lead to death. Whether an individual chooses to adhere to the unwritten rules about healthy behaviours in order not to threaten the existence of the relationship or whether informal sanctions are imposed, the result is often the same. A form of control appears to prevent married people from indulging in risky lifestyles.

Closely related to the explanation that marriage can control behaviour in a positive way is the explanation that marriage is a social relationship that has a stabilizing influence. Being married may facilitate an orderly lifestyle.[111] If risky lifestyles are a threat to health, eating regular meals, getting regular sleep and holding a job are the flip side of the coin, representing the more routine patterns of living that help keep people well.

Much of this considerable research into social relationships has stemmed from evidence that unmarried individuals have higher death rates. The fundamental explanation has been that social isolation is bad. Stated more positively, when individuals are integrated into society (in this case by marriage) they gain a sense of meaning and purpose which in turn affects their motivations and lifestyles.[112] But a whole new set of explanations is needed for the disquieting fact that higher death rates for the unmarried are even more pronounced for men than for women.[113] If social relationships play a part in keeping us alive, men may be more vulnerable to the disruption of those relationships, including marriage.

The greater vulnerability for men (and greater risk of death) has a great deal to do with how the benefits and sacrifices of marriage are divided. Early research in the area of mortality and marital status concluded that women derived fewer of the benefits offered by marriage than men did.[114] In these earlier studies women reported they conformed to society's expectation of their submissive role, often with harm to their own identity. They also found the day-to-day activities of a housewife constricted and frustrating. A new generation, however, may be experiencing a different power structure in marriage as women seek more rewarding roles.

Even the social support benefit of marriage is not always equally divided. Women are more likely to maintain various alternative sources of social support outside of marriage, such as a confidant other than a spouse.[115] In fact, one study of middle-aged women in Massachusetts found that approximately a third of the married women did not mention their husbands at all as members of their support network.[116]

We have only to look at what happens when someone loses their marriage partner through death to see how men and women differ in their abilities to cope without the social support they once had. Feelings of depression are so much a part of the emotion of grief that they are considered a normal reaction and we are not surprised to find such feelings when a loved one is lost. What is surprising, however, is that studies have shown widowed males more depressed than widowed females.[117] And besides their higher rates of depression, widowers have higher rates of more serious mental illness than the rates for widows, a level of mental illness that might require admission to psychiatric hospitals or outpatient clinics.

Health in general suffers in widowhood. Besides depression and mental illness, rates of physical illness are greater for widowed people than for those who are married. They consult physicians more often, consume more drugs, and generally have more symptoms of illness. Within these higher rates, the rates for widowers are higher again than for widows. Rate differences for mortality are also more significant; widowers are at higher risk than widows. Studies have shown them to have highest mortality compared to widows for liver cirrhosis, homicide, and motor vehicle accidents, and only slight lower for tuberculosis and suicide.

These findings of various research studies underline both the negative consequences of partner loss and the more serious consequences for men. If the disappearance of a partner's personal support is the key, as researchers have also shown, why are men less likely than women to find alternative sources of support? The answers are speculation, but because the guesses are made by men as often as women they are worth examining. It has been suggested that men are less willing to admit to feelings of loneliness during separation or bereavement; it could even be less socially acceptable for them to do so. To admit to a need for companionship may be just as difficult. These feelings are not normally compatible with our images of male-ness and self-sufficiency. On a more practical level, during marriage men may have become relatively more isolated from social contacts outside work. They are more likely to rely exclusively on their wives as confidants. They are also more likely to rely on their wives to carry out the job of developing, nurturing, and maintaining other social contacts for them both as a married couple. When separation or widowhood strikes, such skills are already in place for women and sadly lacking for men.

Widowed men also fare worse than widowed women in their ability to go on living without the informal social controls of marriage, including orderly lifestyles and compliance with healthy behaviours.[118] It has been suggested that men may benefit more from the stabilizing influence of marriage where patterns of eating, sleeping, working, and playing are maintained, as well as from the reduction of risk-taking behaviour and the motivation to look after their health.

While lack of social support has been consistently identified as a primary reason for higher death rates for the unmarried, there are competing explanations. The drop in income at marriage dissolution may play a part; it is now generally acknowledged that a lack of material resources can be detrimental to health and long life, as will be shown in the next section. The causes could also be reversed. Illness in separation or widowhood could cause a drop in income. While lack of material resources may be associated with higher death rates for the unmarried, however, it fails to explain why men are more seriously affected, given their comparatively higher incomes in every country where such information is recorded.

Another competing explanation is that married people live longer because people who are likely to live long are also likely to marry. This explanation entails a selection process when individuals seek a mate, a process in which the winners are the fit and the losers are the not so fit. If such selection does take place, it is at best only a partial explanation. Among the losers, men still have higher death rates than women for reasons that clearly have nothing to do with selection.

The role of social support in keeping married death rates below unmarried death rates remains the most consistent explanation, and there is some logic to the suggestion that men are more in need of such social supports than women are. These conclusions about an association between marital status and mortality may apply across most causes of death, but the association is strongest for those causes where behaviour and psychological state play a substantial role (for example, liver cirrhosis and suicide) and weakest for diseases where they have minimal influence, such as some cancers. As a result, the contribution to the gap between male and female life expectancies is difficult to measure. The association is best considered an indirect cause of some of the unhealthy behaviours that are risk factors for the leading causes of death.

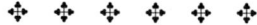

Cutting across the widowed, divorced, married, and never-married is the connection between mortality and social class. The finding in several countries that lower socioeconomic groups have higher death rates than upper socioeconomic groups, regardless of marital status, demonstrates that some of the protective effects of marriage must be economic in nature. Following divorce there is usually substantial economic loss for women; following death of a partner, both men and women can suffer economically.

Studies of death rates as they relate to income, education, occupational level, or all three, have been conducted in the last two decades in Canada, England and Wales, the U.S., France, Germany, Hungary, Sweden, Norway, Denmark, Finland, New Zealand, and Japan. In the process, and despite differences of method in determining socioeconomic status, the general conclusions of medical and social researchers have converged.

A 1993 study by an American team is one of the more recent.[119] Using published data from a national mortality study of those who died in 1960 and 1986, researchers divided a large sample from each year into sub-groups representing different levels of income and education, or socioeconomic status. Information on income and education was obtained from census data and from questionnaires completed by next of kin. For both 1960 and 1986 the research team found a strong association between socioeconomic status and mortality—the lower the socioeconomic status, the higher the mortality. In other words, poor or poorly educated persons had higher death rates than wealthier or better educated persons. A comparison of the 1960 results with the later results of 1986 revealed further disturbing information: the differences in death rates between the poor and non-poor increased during the 26 years of the study and this growing gap occurred while general mortality declined in the U.S. and all other countries of the world. Although death rates were improving for the population as a whole, the benefits were clearly not shared equally.

Another American team examined the relationship between mortality and the equality with which income is distributed in the U.S.[120] To measure income inequality, researchers calculated the percentage of a state's total income received by the poorest half of the state's households. This percentage for each of 50 states was calculated for 1980 and 1990 and compared with each state's mortality rate in those years. The findings indicated that the proportion of a state's total income received by the poorest 50 percent was significantly related to mortality. States with greater inequality in the distribution of income had higher death rates, and this relationship was stronger for 1990 than for 1980. A similar study conducted in Canada in 1992 showed no relationship between income inequality and mortality in ten provinces.[121] Researchers speculated that publicly-funded health care may exempt Canada from the negative effects found in the U.S.

Other developed countries have shown the same pattern as that of the U.S. study. Japan, with the most egalitarian income distribution of any country on record, has the highest life expectancy. In 12 European countries a comparison of changes in income distribution between 1975 and 1985 showed a very close relationship between improvements in income equality and improvements in life expectancy.[122]

In Britain researchers calculated income levels for a wide range of male occupations and compared them with corresponding mortality rates.[123] Comparisons over a 20-year period revealed a strong association between changes in mortality and occupational earnings. As wages rose, death rates declined. A study of the elderly receiving British government pensions also revealed that, over a period of 17 years, death rates declined as the value of pensions increased.

The World Health Organization reports that several other studies have been undertaken in developed countries.[124] A longitudinal study in France covering 500,000 men and an equal number of women showed the lowest mortality for professors and executives and the highest mortality for labourers, whose death rates were three times as high as those of professors. A comparison of mortality among German males aged 30 to 69 in the city of Stuttgart also found that the highest mortality level occurred among unskilled workers. In New Zealand social class differences in mortality were investigated with similar results—lower class mortality rates were approximately twice those of the highest class (with social class defined from high to low as professional and managerial occupations, intermediate occupations, skilled, partly skilled, and unskilled occupations). With roughly the same age group and social class definitions, the results of a study in Finland showed an increasing level of mortality from the higher social group of upper white-collar workers to the group of unskilled workers. The Finnish study also found the differences more pronounced among men than women. In Japan, where a similar study was undertaken, the lowest death rates among males aged 15 and over were reported for managers and the highest rates for miners and the unemployed.

Several Canadian studies provide evidence that lower income is related to higher mortality in Canada, as it is in other countries. Hirdes and Forbes, mentioned earlier in relation to marital status, examined socioeconomic status and mortality among 2,000 45-year-old Ontario males by conducting annual interviews with study participants for almost 20 years. The results demonstrated that low-income men had a higher risk of mortality than higher-income men. Earlier research studies conducted by Health and Welfare Canada focused on the same relationship in metropolitan areas, accounting for roughly 60 percent of the Canadian population.[125] Census tract information on income from census years 1971 and 1986 was compared with corresponding mortality rates, with results showing substantially greater life expectancies in the highest income quintiles. Other research examined mortality among Canadian native people (whose incomes fall dramatically below average Canadian incomes) and found a disproportionately high level of mortality.[126]

Canadian research has also focused on male-female differences in the effects of income on death rates. Health and Welfare Canada studies found that the importance of income level was significantly greater for men than for women. The differences in life expectancy between the highest and lowest income levels in 1971 were 6.2 years for males and 2.9 years for females. By 1986 the differences had decreased to 5.6 and 1.8 respectively. Within low-income levels the greater mortality for men was especially apparent for cancer, diseases of the circulatory system, accidents, and respiratory diseases, the leading causes of death.

In light of such conclusive findings throughout the developed world, there have been a number of theories offered to explain why poverty should affect mortality. A practical explanation suggested by American researchers has been that without adequate resources, the poor are unable to purchase health insurance and unable to adopt a healthy lifestyle, especially by purchasing the proper foods for a healthy diet. In support of this, one study found a strong relationship between a state's level of income inequality and the number of people receiving food stamps and the number without health insurance.[127]

Poor nutrition in general was identified by researchers in both the U.K. and the U.S. as a reason for higher death rates of the poor. The British study of pensioners calculated the statistical association between life expectancy and several measures of food and nutrients. It found strong positive correlations with consumption of vitamin C, vitamin A, and green vegetables. On the other hand, consumption of carbohydrates showed a negative correlation. While the nutrition connection with life expectancy was strong, it may be a mistake to assume that inadequate nutrition of the poor plays a large part in the association between low income and life expectancy. A study of mortality risk factors in Japan found that green vegetables reduce the mortality rate not only at lower incomes but at all income levels. At the same time, meat consumption shifted the mortality rate upward, again across the board. In light of these more general associations, the researcher[128] concluded that risk factors like poor nutrition had their impact on mortality quite independent of socioeconomic status.

It has also been argued that poor housing and poor neighbourhoods contribute to the increased mortality for low-income groups. While the relationship with poor housing is difficult to measure or test, it remains a popular explanation. Nonetheless, the British study on pensioners showed that their relative expenditures on housing failed to explain the association between pension levels and death rates, once smoking and inadequate nutrition were taken out of the equation. Poor neighbourhoods, on the other hand, provide a better explanation, according to several researchers. For example, the American study examining the effect of income inequality on mortality in all 50 states found that states with greater inequality had higher rates of homicide, other violent crimes, and per capita expenditure on police protection, factors generally associated with poor neighbourhoods.

Poor nutrition, poor housing, and poor neighbourhoods are all indicators of class differences in living standards. The living standards of the poor improved over the last quarter of the twentieth century in developed countries, but differences still remain. It has been argued that even with this improvement, it is not the absolute standard of living that is important in life expectancy but the levels of isolation, self-esteem, and anxiety that accompany relative poverty.[129] These are more in the nature of psychological outcomes of poverty at the individual level. Still, at their root are the broader social characteristics that separate the classes, such as differences in nutrition, housing, and neighbourhoods.

While research evidence points to factors beyond the control of the poor, such as their inability to afford proper nutrition, a less violent neighbourhood, or medical attention, there is also evidence of lifestyle choices that may be considered within their control. Smoking is the most obvious. The study of pensioners in Britain found tobacco to be one of the most significant expenditures in explaining the association between income and mortality.[130] The Canadian study of 21 census metropolitan areas also attributed a good portion of the gap in death rates between higher and lower income groups to smoking. In particular, differences in death rates for heart disease, stroke, and lung cancer grew larger as income level declined, especially for men. The gap varied only slightly or was non-existent for women. These findings were consistent with other Canadian research information on the major risk factors for these causes of death. Regular cigarette smoking in Canada has historically been more prevalent among males. In addition, regular smoking is more prevalent for both sexes among lower income groups.[131]

In looking for explanations it is clear there are more theories than proof. Despite general agreement about the relationship between income and mortality there is little agreement about why this is so. Moreover, few researchers have ventured to guess why men are more affected than women. The Canada Health and Welfare study is an exception, with its identification of smoking as the primary cause of the male-female difference. But few studies have looked into whether, among the poor, men are more likely to experience lower standards of nutrition or to live in poorer housing and poorer neighborhoods than women.

Even without knowing why, however, social class has a significant effect on life expectancy and the effect is greater for men, as Canadian studies have shown. These gender differences have to be added to the more pronounced effects of marital status on men's life expectancies than on women's. In fact, men get more than a double dose of impact from these two risk factors. An interesting 1994 study of 20,000 American adults between 25 and 74 years of age showed that unmarried status and poverty interact—even feed each other—to create an especially harmful force that diminishes health.[132] On top of this, their joint effects are even more harmful for men, although the reasons are still not known. Looking at it more positively, Canadian researchers Hirdes and Forbes estimate that the cumulative effects of high social support found in marriage, high income, and being a non-smoker can provide an 18-fold reduction in the risk of mortality for men.

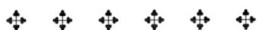

Society can be neatly divided into male and female, old and young, married and unmarried, and high, medium, and low income groups. The availability of information on such categories in the public record or in research studies of large experimental groups makes the testing of their association with mortality easier. As a result they have undergone considerable testing, enough to build a consensus that among these non-lifestyle risk factors those with the greatest risk are old age, male sex, low income, and unmarried status.

Society is also divided into geographical areas and this category too has an effect on mortality. In world society a female infant in Japan, for example, can expect to live on average 82 years and a male infant, 76 years. In Uganda, on the other hand, a female infant can expect to live 42 years and a male, 40 years. Canada ranks high in international comparisons, with a life expectancy of 81 for women and 75 for men in 1997. These international variations inevitably lead to a search for reasons, and the consensus has been that living standards, diet, and lifestyle have been contributing factors.

Within Canada death rates vary regionally. Age-standardized death rates which adjust for local variations in age distribution are highest in the Atlantic provinces and lowest in the western provinces. Income levels explain some of these differences. The impact of diet and nutrition (green vegetables, vitamin A, vitamin C, unsaturated fats) is not so easily measured; national studies of fruit and vegetable consumption in the 1990s did not identify significant regional differences. Given the time lag between risk factors and the development of lifestyle diseases, the effects of smoking and alcohol abuse are also difficult to measure. The association of death rates with smoking rates 20 years ago has been mentioned earlier (in chapter 4). Today smoking rates are high in the Atlantic provinces and Quebec, low in British Columbia, and close to the national average in other provinces, but these rates will affect mortality years from now. Internal migration also plays a role. According to Statistics Canada, in the first half of the 1990s close to a quarter of Canadians moved from one city to another, sometimes to a city in a different province, making it difficult to determine where an individual was exposed to risk factors that might end in disease later.

Countries are also made up of urban and rural areas. A recent U.S. study examined the impact of urban residence on mortality and found the mortality risk of city residents almost twice as high as that of rural or small town residents, regardless of their marital status, education, or income.[133] Gender, however, made a difference; the high mortality risk of urban residence was significant only for men. In addition, the mortality risk differences were not as significant among those older than 65.

Because the study found mortality risk in cities most significant for two causes of death, infections and tumours, the authors commented that the elevated levels of tumour deaths suggested the influence of physical, chemical, and biological exposures in urban areas. Living in cities also involves the stress of noise, sensory stimulation to the point of overload, interpersonal relations and conflict, and vigilance against crime and accidents. These can be found at home or at work or at places in between. While such examples of stress are more prevalent in the city, the city may not be the place that can provide the necessary social supports to deal with them.

Urban living is yet another factor affecting life expectancy, and can be added to other risk factors that explain the gap between men and women. Why women do not appear to experience the same increased risk of urban living is not certain. Researchers speculated that men may spend more time in work or other environments that are risky to health, yet their data showed that the employment or occupation status of study participants made no difference to the outcome. This finding also puts into question their speculation that elevated levels of tumour deaths may be caused by more physical, chemical, or biological exposures in urban areas, especially when city women were surely experiencing the same exposures. Their findings show instead that smoking and drinking, not employment or occupation, may have made the impact of city residence worse for study participants, especially men. In fact, the impact was largely absent for those younger than 65 years who neither drank nor had ever smoked. A large role for these behavioural risk factors seems a more logical conclusion to draw from elevated levels of tumour deaths.

Chapter 8

Years of Life Lost

There are other ways to look at the impact on society of shorter lifespans for men. Besides comparing mortality rates of men and women, health researchers have also estimated the potential years of life lost when an individual dies prematurely. In Canada years of life lost are generally the difference between the age of actual death and an average life expectancy of 75 (in the 1990s). For the major causes of death, years of life lost are greater for men than for women—three and a half times greater for heart disease, three times greater for motor vehicle accidents and suicide, and over one and a half times greater for lung cancer.

Because men have lower rates of chronic illness in their later years than women do, these potential lost years are for the most part *healthy* years. If premature death is by accident or suicide, half a lifetime of healthy years could be lost. If death is the result of lifestyle diseases, the lost years are nearly always chopped off the leisure years, the last fifth of a lifetime when work and family responsibilities are at an end. Both men and women have earned that social reward, that period referred to by Browning in his hopeful lines:

Grow old along with me!
The best is yet to be,
The last of life, for which the first was made.

For many men, however, the end of responsibility is followed too soon by the end of life. By any measure, it is a tragic waste.

Estimates show that over a million potential years of male life were lost in a single year in the 1990s in Canada.[134] It would be interesting—if not heartbreaking—to know something of the male lives that preceded those lost years. For every man who died prematurely, how much of his heart and soul went into building a relationship with a marriage partner; how many tears and doubts went into raising his children and preparing them for independence; how much discipline and financial sacrifice went into making it possible to finally quit work? This is the real work of a lifetime. When the rewards come at the end, you want to be alive to enjoy them.

Estimates of years lost miss the human dimension of years spent. Case histories may serve the purpose better, and four are presented here. The reader who is more comfortable with statistics might prefer to skip this chapter.

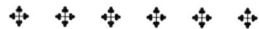

Fifty years ago in postwar Canada young people were making up for lost time by looking for partners for the long term as the future began to hold more promise. Joan and Gordon were two such young people, although neither of them would have thought of themselves as players in a typical case history.

When Joan and Gordon first began to date in their mid-twenties, Joan's friends predicted the relationship would last a month, while his friends gave it a week. The difference of a few weeks was probably nothing more than the higher degree of cynicism among Gordon's friends who, recently finishing their university education through government grants for war veterans, were beginning their careers in the relatively new world of advertising, a business based on a cynical view of our willingness to be manipulated into buying products we don't need. Motivational research was reaching new heights of respectability, and no one was more amused by its meteoric rise than account executives of advertising agencies. No, the similarity in the predictions of Gordon's friends and Joan's friends was more significant than the difference. Everyone agreed they wouldn't last. They were at opposite poles of every possible measure of personality.

Gordon played the game of keeping up appearances while Joan

was sometimes a bit unpolished and, what was worse, resisted all attempts by friends to take off the rough edges, just as she had resisted her parents' attempts for years. In all things he was a pessimist; she, an optimist. He was carefree about money; she was overly careful. As if personality differences weren't enough, Gordon was from eastern Canada; Joan, from the west. He was a Roman Catholic; she, a Protestant.

Almost as if to prove everyone wrong, they had a short courtship and married three months from their first date (in a Catholic Church ceremony).

And so began almost fifty years of getting to know each other, after the fact. In Gordon's view, a wife and family had an important role to play in his life. They were to be the stabilizing factor through the ups and downs of the competitive business world he was in. His wife would be there to listen; his two sons were to excel at school and sports. His perfect family would be a reflection of his own personal success.

For Joan's part, marriage and family gave her the opportunity to be a hostess/mother/gardener/gourmet cook/community-activist all rolled into one. Gordon's needs and her needs could all be accommodated in her vision of a family.

On their tenth anniversary they told friends they had a happy marriage. She had gone out to work and he was about to trade in a rocky career in the advertising business for regular hours and a steadier income in the government. They had adjusted to some truths about themselves and each other—his carefree attitude about money didn't make a good fit with job insecurity and her roles as hostess and gourmet cook were a disaster (she performed poorly at both).

They made other discoveries as the years went by. Their respect for each other's needs was not always forthcoming. While they seethed and smarted about such failures from time to time, they tried to concentrate on their common goal—happiness and success for their two sons—a goal that was not always evident to their children, especially as they struggled through adolescence.

Money management became increasingly important and a

constant source of tension as the university years began. It seemed there was always enough money for someone to clean the house and prepare meals while Joan worked but never enough for a more prestigious car or membership in a better tennis club. On their 25th anniversary Joan and Gordon told friends they had a happy marriage, despite rumours that they were splitting.

The two boys left home one after another to make their way on their own. Surprisingly, their parents seemed to blossom in the empty nest. Money matters began to take a back seat; the mortgage was paid off and they talked about a better car. There were weddings and babies over the next few years, and Joan and Gordon confided in each other that their new role as grandparents gave them all the pleasures of seeing young children occasionally and none of the responsibilities. They began to plan for Gordon's retirement—ski holidays and bicycle tours they had dreamed about for years. On their 40th anniversary they told friends they were never more in love.

Only a few of their dream vacations came about, however. Returning from a ski holiday in March one year Gordon felt sick enough to make a rare doctor's appointment. Joan was sure he'd let himself get overtired, but x-rays and other tests followed in short order with devastating results. He had lung cancer, very likely connected to a smoking habit that had ended fifteen years earlier. Gordon died at the age of 70 and, without her partner of 45 years, Joan began a long period of living on her own with a mixture of sadness and bitterness. According to health statistics, five years of Gordon's life was lost. Even without the statistics, it was as if he had run a grueling marathon and received his prize posthumously.

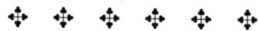

Another case history illustrates that the marathon is not always run at an even pace. Even erratic progress is hard work, with the added pressure of finishing before time runs out.

It is true that heredity has a role in our personal development—genes can predispose us to certain behaviour patterns. But according to experts in the field of developmental psychology, there appears to be a larger role for events in our childhood and subsequent growing years. Louis could attest to this, although he never realized it himself and never gained enough insight into how his childhood had affected him to gain a good level of self-awareness.

A beautiful infant and a quiet, agreeable toddler, he was the object of his parents' devotion and the centre of their universe. This was the environment of security and affection he lived in until he was two years of age when his parents, expecting their second child, sent him to live with his grandparents in another province. Whether this drastic measure resulted from misguided medical advice or from his parents' desire to replace him with someone better was never made clear to him.

Louis returned to his family over a year later. There would be many years of searching for the personality he believed would win back the place he held in his parents' hearts before he was sent away. It seemed logical to invent something new, and he did. Finally childhood was left behind. In his adolescence Louis was everyone's idea of the young man "most likely to succeed"—he was good-looking, confident, outgoing, and known for his sense of humour. Or so it seemed on the surface.

When Nicole first began to date him he was all those things and more. Just recently discharged from the army at war's end, he had a certain worldliness about him that civilian 21-year-olds were lacking. Not only that, young Canadians were no different than young people in other countries recently at war. They were going to the altar in record numbers. As soon as Louis found a job, he and Nicole were married.

It wasn't long before Louis' doubts about himself began to surface, especially in the work world. The outgoing personality turned out to be a manufactured object, something that had served him well in adolescence, but was more difficult to maintain as the years went on. Drinking and after-hours partying with work colleagues was a good way of carrying on the myth of self-confidence, but it began to interfere with job performance. In the years that followed job tenures became shorter, sometimes Louis' idea, sometimes his employer's. He moved Nicole and his family to other cities in search of employment, four times in all.

Despite the problems and pressures, there were few periods of unemployment. Five children were fed, clothed, and educated over 25 years. While part of Louis was taking on these adult responsibilities, however, part of him was still stuck in adolescence. The never-ending pressure to provide for his family kept him from sorting out this major discrepancy.

The jolt to his self-delusion came when he and Nicole separated after 30 years of marriage. Nicole had had enough. Then followed Louis' struggle to overcome the demons that had plagued him, not a steady progression toward improvement but, after several setbacks, an overall climb into self-awareness. The children had grown and left home in the meantime. Louis and Nicole decided to try again—they were still in their 60s and there were many years ahead to make things work. Louis made better progress after their reconciliation; he began to find his true personality again. But the damage of heavy drinking over the years was beyond permanent repair. He died of heart disease at the age of 71. He hadn't given up the struggle for maturity and personal identity. He simply ran out of time.

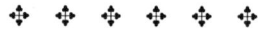

Derrick shook hands with his tennis opponent at the end of another match of straight sets. He played an aggressive game of tennis that overpowered the top players in the club in every annual tournament. One admiring competitor claimed he had never seen Derrick play a safe shot in his life. Long base-line rallies were not for him; he was up at the net whenever he could possibly put the point away. And many times when it was foolhardy to even try.

In other areas of his life Derrick was just as successful. Starting as early as his high school years, he had excelled at sports. He had also shown a remarkable talent for starting projects with nothing but his own savings and turning them into profitable ventures. After a day of caddying at a local golf course, he would spent the night retrieving abandoned balls for resale, finally paying a friend an hourly rate to help him. During the school year he charged a small fee for a school newsletter he produced on his computer. That particular project, which soon involved a paid staff of three, netted him enough to start his own soft drink vending business at one of the area beaches in the summer.

When high school and university years were over, he went to work for an investment firm. He was responsible for most of the acquisitions his firm made over the next ten years, putting to work the skills he had learned in his own enterprises. At forty years of age, he was thinking of going out on his own.

The idea of setting up his own business had begun to hatch only three months earlier, when one of his children had been diagnosed with a rare medical disorder. Derrick and his wife Tracey were devastated by the news. It immobilized them for weeks before they forced themselves to talk about it and plan for the future, despite the pain of facing reality. The most pessimistic medical opinion was that the child, a boy, would live only five more years; the most optimistic, that he might grow to young adulthood before he died. There was also a frightening wait-and-see prognosis with the other two children who were too young for reliable testing.

The earliest decision was that Tracey would resign her job and care for her son personally. Derrick could also become more involved if his time were his own, but the demands of his firm were considerable. After a great deal of discussion, Tracey and Derrick's second decision was that he would go out on his own. It was, in fact, Derrick's proposal made with his usual confidence about any risks involved and with a growing feeling that he could even do better financially if the rewards of his hard work came to him directly. He had another reason for wanting more time outside work. He wanted to begin researching his son's illness, looking for new developments anywhere in the world, and perhaps finding one or two with promise. With his energy and ability to get things done, he could spearhead an aggressive campaign for more research funding for this relatively rare illness. He could use his knowledge of tax laws to sell some of the many contacts he had in the business world and he might be able to find his way around the government research network and get additional funding there. Tennis and golf would have to be put aside. For the first time in his life he realized how valuable his children were to him.

As they set about their most important project together, Tracey was never more proud of her husband. He spent half of each day in his new investment business and half in research. The funding contacts would come later. In the middle of this atmosphere of activity, an invitation to the wind-up dinner at the tennis club arrived, announcing a major presentation to Derrick for a record number of club championships. They both agreed he would have to attend alone while Tracey looked after the children.

At the dinner there seemed to be an unending number of toasts to Derrick's achievement, and when the evening was over there seemed to be just as many offers to drive him home. It was true he had been drinking more than usual, but there had been too many years of handling challenges successfully to consider this as anything but one more challenge. He waved off the offers of a drive. He placed his championship cup on the back seat of his car and turned on to the familiar two-lane highway that would take him ten miles to home. When he pulled out to pass a minivan a minute later he saw oncoming lights. They were far enough away, he estimated, for him to make it easily. But he had underestimated the speed of the oncoming car and at the last second had to swerve off the road to avoid a head-on collision. At home Tracey paced and worried for hours before they reached her with the tragic news. She had lost a husband and father who was trying to do so much for his family. Health researchers could have translated it into numbers for her. Thirty-five potential years of life had been lost.

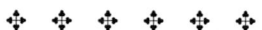

Cheryl hadn't really been looking for a husband. She'd been looking for a father for her children, yet to be born, and she would marry him only if he insisted. Today such an arrangement might not turn anyone's head, but in the 1950s Cheryl was considered a little strange. Nonetheless on those terms she found Cameron, who seemed to have the requisite set of genes to pass on to beautiful, intelligent, athletic, even-tempered children. He agreed to father three children for Cheryl but insisted on marriage. After much negotiation, he had his way.

As each baby arrived, friends and relatives marvelled at the success of Cheryl's project. The two male infants were good-looking, the female quite beautiful. As the years went on, however, one boy was a little slow at school, the other not so coordinated athletically, and the girl had a quick temper. Still the pluses were greater than the minuses.

The largest plus of all was the fact that Cameron and Cheryl's marriage appeared to be made in heaven. He found her strange ways always exciting and she found him a steady provider and someone who agreed with her that children were the be-all and end-all of life. Despite all threats and persuasion, however, she couldn't get him to end his smoking habit, and by the time the children were in their teenage years, Cameron had developed a persistent cough.

Family holidays were the highlight of every year. When the children were very small, camping was hard work for Cameron and Cheryl. But as they grew, the children took over most of the chores at the campground and continued to accompany their parents each summer, right into their late teens. Cameron had indeed turned out to be the perfect father, not only because he shared his near-perfect genes but because he was patient and loving, teaching them to swim, canoe, sail, fish, and respect wild life.

By the time his grandchildren came along Cameron began to look forward to teaching them the same skills. His coughing and shortness of breath, which had been diagnosed as bronchitis, were now a major handicap in all the activities he wanted to be a part of with the newest generation of children. At 55, he decided to give up smoking. With a great deal of reinforcement from Cheryl and the family he was successful. He found he could swim farther, paddle longer, and carry children more easily. The doctor warned that some of the past damage to his lungs was permanent, but Cameron enjoyed even the modest improvement in his breathing.

Over the next several years he began to talk of retiring early. With some careful planning, he and Cheryl could start up a wilderness camping program for children in the provincial park. They began their plans enthusiastically but Cheryl was the first to notice that Cameron tired easily and was still bothered by laboured breathing. The doctor moved him on to new medication which gave him some temporary relief. There was hope that his post-retirement plans for full summers out of the city would reduce exposure to environmental pollutants and help him even more.

But it became increasingly evident that it was too late. Cameron's health deteriorated rapidly and, after a few weeks in the hospital during which he complained about missing a particularly beautiful camping season, he died at the age of 68, the perfect father of three and the perfect grandfather of eight.

At the funeral service one grandchild, eight years old, delivered his own personal eulogy, claiming that his grandfather had promised to teach him how to make a birchbark canoe when he got out of the hospital. Now he was gone, taking all the wonderful things he knew with him and taking them too soon.

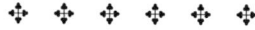

Precious years of life are lost when someone dies prematurely. In four typical case histories, a total of 46 years of life were lost after hopeful plans had been laid to make the years worthwhile. Like the grandchild struggling to understand, one is left wondering why those who went too soon were in such a hurry to go.

CHAPTER 9

Gender Differences, Widening and Narrowing

In recording mortality trends worldwide, the United Nations divides the world into developed countries (more recently called developed market economies by the UN) and developing countries. In between is a small group of countries called economies in transition, primarily former socialist countries of Europe that made up the U.S.S.R. Many developing countries are still at the stage of high mortality as developed countries were at the beginning of the twentieth century, and many economies in transition are at the mortality levels of the developed countries in the 1960s.

Despite these slower advances for some, mortality rates in most countries of the world are dropping, though at different rates. The largest gains in life expectancy are now being made in developing countries. These gains have been made as a result of the availability of medical tools to combat infectious diseases, which have been the major causes of death in those countries. By the end of the century developing countries were beginning to win the battle, but infectious diseases still caused roughly 42 percent of all deaths compared to 47 percent attributed to non-communicable diseases. (The remaining 11 percent of deaths were the result of accidents.) With infectious diseases still taking a heavy toll in developing countries, life expectancies remained low. Most African and Asian countries in this category had life expectancies in the 50s and 60s in 1995, while those of a good number of countries were still in the 40s. Exceptions were a few Latin American countries with life expectancies in the low 70s.

As mortality rates drop in developing countries females have moved slightly ahead of males in life expectancy. Until recently this was not the case. As in western countries in the nineteenth and earlier centuries, women in Asia and Africa carried a large physical burden in local economies along with the hazards of less advanced childbirth methods and the responsibilities of child care. For the most part, their lifespans were shorter than men's. As women gained the longevity advantage, the gap between their lifespans and those of men remained small (ranging from two to five years) in the last twenty years of the twentieth century. During this period three-quarters of those countries recorded by the United Nations showed no change. The tendency of the gap to remain small is not surprising, given the large part that was still played by childbirth deaths in mortality figures. The next twenty years, however, are expected to tell a different story. Researchers for the World Health Organization predict the male-female gap in developing countries will widen as a result of changing lifestyles in many of these countries;[135] in a few South American countries like Brazil and Chile the gap has already started to widen.

The decline in the proportion of infectious diseases and the growth in the proportion of non-communicable diseases will be responsible for the widening gap, repeating the pattern of developed countries over the twentieth century. Most of the major non-communicable diseases, which have become known as lifestyle diseases, take a larger toll on men, who show a greater tendency than women to choose risky lifestyles, as earlier chapters have shown. In particular, World Health Organization researchers attribute the widening gap to the so-called tobacco epidemic that has spread in developing countries over the past two decades.

In countries with economies in transition, such as Russia, Ukraine, Poland and others, mortality caused by infectious diseases declined in the postwar period. Today life expectancies are 10 to 15 years longer than those of developing countries, 70 for Poland, Albania, Bulgaria, and Lithuania being typical. There have been setbacks, however, along the way toward longer lifespans. As the proportion of non-communicable diseases in economies in transition increased in the 1960s, mortality from cardiovascular diseases remained consistently high and several countries lost ground in life expectancy, especially among males. According to UN demographic experts, the high prevalence of high-risk behaviour (including smoking and excessive alcohol intake) and the high fat content of the diet typical of countries with economies in transition were major factors in the stagnating or declining life expectancies of men.[136] By the 1990s some of these countries were showing signs of recovery. Throughout these downward and upward trends, life expectancies for women have been considerably higher than for men, a gap that has widened until it is now in the range of roughly 9 to 12 years. This gap is predicted to widen further during the next 20 years, during which women in economies in transition may gain another four years in life expectancy, while men may barely gain a year.

In developed countries, deaths from infectious diseases now represent only six percent of all deaths on average. They are no longer the major health concern they once were; for over half a century non-communicable diseases have been the main killers. After many years of upward trends in mortality from non-communicable diseases, the major trend emerging in the last quarter of the twentieth century was the decline in rates of mortality from ischemic or coronary heart disease. More recently some developed countries also have shown declines in cancer mortality and mortality from accidents, notably motor vehicle accidents. Because heart disease has led the way in total numbers of deaths its decline in particular has significantly lowered mortality in general, and the cancer and accident declines will soon begin to have an influence as well. Over the last two decades life expectancy in developed countries has shown an overall gain of five years.

Moreover, the decline in heart disease mortality has been slightly greater for men than for women, even more so in the case of accidents, and the later decline in cancer mortality has been mainly restricted to men, all three trends affecting the male-female gap in life expectancy. As a result, while the gap has just begun to appear in developing countries and is widening in economies in transition, it appears to have reached a peak in several developed countries.

Among 22 countries in this category, the gap has begun to level off since the 1980s in seven and has even narrowed in eleven.[137] In the early 1980s Canada's longevity gap, for example, was seven years; by the 1990s it was six. In the U.S. it also dropped, though slightly (from 7.4 years to 6.8 years), and in the U.K. it dropped from six to five years.

Despite the narrowing of the longevity gap in 11 developed countries, the World Health Organization predicts that life expectancy for women will grow more rapidly than for men over the next 20 years with lifestyle factors still playing a part in mortality in these countries. If these predictions become reality, the current narrowing of the gap between men and women will have proven to be an aberration. It is too early to say. Nonetheless, it may be useful to explore the underlying reasons for the current narrowing whether it is here to stay or not.

It is significant that the peak in the longevity gap in the 1980s followed on the heels of the peak in heart disease mortality. That they are now coming down concurrently is also significant. When death rates from heart disease were at their peak in the late 1970s and early 1980s, heart disease was the leading cause of death in developed countries, and it took the lives of twice as many men as women. These two characteristics of heart disease—a high mortality rate and a high male-female ratio—made it one of the main villains in the gap between men's and women's life expectancies. Just how large a role it played was shown in a United Nations study carried out during those peak years. To determine the share of the damage that should be attributed to heart disease (and other causes of death), the study involved statistical calculations that took into account mortality rates, age distribution, and sex mortality ratios by cause of death in each country.[138] Findings revealed that heart disease made the largest contribution to the differences in life expectancy, contributing an estimated two years of the average difference of seven years. Not only did heart disease have a large impact on the longevity gap, but its long steady growth leading up to its peak was credited with having more influence than all other factors combined on the fact that men's life expectancy fell increasingly behind women's as the century progressed.[139]

Within a decade, the gap in some developed countries—including Canada—would begin to narrow. Given its predominant role in widening the gap earlier, it is not surprising to find heart disease making a large contribution as it narrows. In Canada male death rates for heart disease fell from 338 per 100,000 in 1979 to 182 in 1997. Over the same period death rates for women fell from 171 per 100,000 to 94. Both sexes have benefitted from improved heart disease death rates but clearly male life expectancy has received the largest boost with twice as many men as women failing to die each year as they did previously.

Because heart disease at its peak in Canada and other developed countries contributed two years to the difference between male and female life expectancies, its decline has played a major role in narrowing the same difference over the past 20 years. Its role will diminish as its share of total deaths diminish, but in the early part of the twenty-first century it is still a major player. Its effect is primarily due to the absolute number of fewer deaths from a male-dominated disease, while a decrease in the predominance of males has probably not yet made a large contribution. The sex-ratio decrease is only slight—men are still twice as likely as women to die of heart disease—but there could be a bottom limit to the decline in the female rate, which is already low, while men could continue to make gains for some time to come.

In the UN study looking at the influence of causes of death, accidents were found to be the next largest contributor to the longevity gap. Although accident numbers were far below heart disease numbers, men in developed countries were three times as likely as women to die as a result of accidents. Moreover, the lives taken by accidents at younger ages increased the impact on life expectancy. Accidents, therefore, were shown to contribute one and a third years of the seven-year difference in men's and women's life expectancies.

From the 1970s to the 1990s accidental deaths declined in developed countries. Road traffic fatalities, the leading cause of accidental death, showed a dramatic decrease. In Canada male mortality for accidents of all categories decreased from 73 per 100,000 in 1979 to 38 in 1996. The comparable female decrease was 29 per 100,000 to 18. The decrease for motor vehicle accidents, in particular, has been 50 percent over the period. Greater gains have been made by men and, despite the fewer number of accidental deaths compared to heart disease deaths, the faster mortality decline for men and the younger age group affected (especially for motor vehicle accidents) have together made a contribution to narrowing the longevity gap over the past two decades.

The UN study also found a smaller but still significant contribution to the gap from cancer, another predominantly male cause of death. Across the developed countries before declines began in the 1980s, men were twice as likely as women to die of cancer on average and six times as likely to die of lung cancer (over five times as likely in Canada). Isolating lung cancer specifically, the study found a contribution of close to a year of the seven-year gap.

Lung cancer mortality rates have now started to decrease in some developed countries. In Canada male rates dropped from 81 per 100,000 in 1988, when they peaked, to 70 in 1998, a surprising decrease of 14 percent in just ten years after rapid growth over the previous fifty. Even more surprising is the fact that female mortality rates have not shown the same decrease but have instead gone up, rising 22 percent, in fact, during the same period. In other words, while both male and female lung cancer rates increased during the 1980s, only female rates continued to increase during the 1990s. This decline in a male-dominated cause of death combined with a dramatic decline in male predominance (helped considerably by female increases) is having an impact on the longevity gap that will bring male and female life expectancies closer together. On the other hand, the impact has been felt for barely a decade and unlikely to be wholly reflected in current life expectancy figures.

Other major contributors to the longevity gap in the past have been respiratory diseases with male-female mortality ratios of 3 to 1 in the 1970s. The chronic diseases of bronchitis, emphysema, and asthma accounted for half a year of the gap, according to the UN study. In Canada chronic respiratory diseases have shown small declines in mortality during the 1990s. Like lung cancer rates, however, there has been improvement for men but no improvement for women, whose mortality rates have, in fact, continued to increase steadily. Male-female ratios are now 1.5 to 1 compared to the ratio of 3 to 1 thirty years ago. Despite these significant changes, the impact on the longevity gap of the male decline in chronic respiratory disease, as with lung cancer, has barely had time to be felt.

If mortality rates for some of the major causes of death are now declining it is good news for life expectancies, especially for men. It would appear that the heart disease decline is having the greatest effect in narrowing the male-female gap, but declines in mortality rates for accidents, lung cancer, and chronic respiratory diseases are also playing a part. Why the rates for these causes of death are going down is the newest challenge for researchers in epidemiology. It has been estimated that most of the decline in heart disease in North America is due to changes in lifestyle.[140] The more recent declines in male death rates for lung cancer, chronic respiratory diseases, and motor vehicle accidents have also been attributed to lifestyle changes for men. Some recent studies have looked at these relationships.

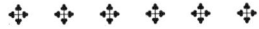

Lifestyles, as distinct from biological factors, account for two-thirds of the longevity gap in developed countries. The myth that, among lifestyles, stressful work has been the primary cause of shorter lives for men for over a century, is still popular. And with the first indication of a narrowing longevity gap, it follows that the quick explanation is usually the new stress experienced by women who have joined the labour force in such large numbers over the past 35 years. Employment for women outside the home, however, has had many beneficial effects on their health and longevity, to be described later in this section.

Much more mundane is the true explanation for the narrowing gap. Between the early 1980s and the early 1990s cigarette consumption declined by 1.5 percent annually in developed countries while it was rising by 1.4 percent annually in developing countries. But women were not well represented in the decline. The prevalence of smoking among women had reached a peak later than the prevalence among men—the 1970s for women as compared with the 1960s for men—and its dire effects on female death rates for lung cancer and chronic respiratory diseases continued (with the usual time lag) even as male death rates were decreasing. At the same time, the delay in female smoking decreases meant slower gains in heart disease declines in the 1980s than those made by men.

When female smoking prevalence finally started to come down in Canada the decreases were barely perceptible in the first years. From 1985 (when Statistics Canada began prevalence studies) to 1991 the decrease was under two percent; men with their earlier start were making much better headway (down 10 percent). From 1991 to 1999, however, women smokers decreased by 13 percent compared to a decrease for men of only 5 percent. Although the overall 14-year decrease of 15 percent was identical for both sexes, the more recent improvements for women have not yet had an impact.

The connection between smoking and the three major causes of death has been shown in earlier chapters. The size and distribution of the connection is revealing. A recent study attributed 15 percent of all deaths in developed countries to tobacco. Roughly a quarter of smoking-related deaths were related to each of ischemic heart disease and lung cancer, and less than an eighth to chronic respiratory diseases.[141] Similar studies undertaken in Canada have been mentioned in Chapter 5. These studies found that a fifth of all deaths in 1996 could be attributed to smoking. Of smoking-related deaths, 30 percent were related to lung cancer, 21 percent to ischemic heart disease, and 16 percent to chronic respiratory diseases.[142] The remaining third were related to various causes of death including other cancers, other heart diseases, stroke, tuberculosis, pneumonia and influenza.

With strong evidence that smoking is connected with death

rates for lung cancer, heart disease, and respiratory diseases, the recent declines in these death rates are being attributed by medical researchers to declines in smoking prevalence for the most part. The decline in smoking for men, while smoking for women continued to rise, has been credited more than any other trend with narrowing the gap between men's and women's life expectancies.

The contribution of alcohol to the recent narrowing of the longevity gap in developed countries is less substantial than the contribution of smoking, but its share is likely considerable. There have simply been less studies of alcohol-attributable deaths. Moreover, the offsetting benefits of moderate alcohol use for heart disease which have come to be recognized have made the net effects of alcohol use difficult to calculate. In contrast to its positive effects on heart disease over the years, alcohol has played a major negative role in traffic accidents. Almost half of all fatally-injured drivers have been drinking. Only in the past 20 years have both alcohol use and traffic fatalities shown declines in the developed world.[143]

The important characteristics of motor vehicle deaths are the very large sex ratio of up to 8 male to 1 female deaths among impaired drivers and the young age groups most affected. These characteristics compensate for the lower death rates for accidents compared to rates for heart disease, lung cancer, and respiratory diseases, and are the principal reasons for their impact on life expectancies.

In Canada alcohol consumption has decreased gradually since the late 1970s, as described in chapter 6. During the same period motor vehicle fatalities have also dropped. While a good portion of fatal accident decreases can be attributed to lower speed limits and automobile safety improvements, health officials also attribute a major portion to reduced drinking resulting from public campaigns designed to encourage more responsible alcohol use. With the number of young lives saved—the overwhelming majority the lives of young men—the decline of alcohol use has helped to move men's life expectancy closer to that of women.

Smoking and alcohol use are twentieth century lifestyles that helped to widen male and female life expectancies and, in turn, helped to narrow them. Other lifestyle changes have taken place during the same period. Consumption of dietary fat, a risk factor for heart disease, has also been declining, but there is no hard evidence that this improvement has been restricted to one sex. For another heart risk factor, work stress, there is also little conclusive evidence that women are disproportionately increasing their risk, but it has been the subject of considerable testing and what one gerontologist has called "energetic discussion."[144] The testing and the discussion have revolved around how women's increasing labour force participation will affect their longevity. A review of the studies related to this controversy may shed some light.

The most recent *Health Report* from Statistics Canada gives the results of national surveys taken in the 1990s of Canadians aged 18 or older. In answer to one of five questions related to stress, roughly 45 percent of women compared to 38 percent of men reported that they were trying to take on too much at once.[145] Followed up four years later, those who reported stress were twice as likely to have developed chronic health conditions such as migraine, ulcers, arthritis, or respiratory diseases as those not reporting stress. Female respondents were more likely to mention respiratory diseases than male respondents. Interestingly, heart disease failed to make this group of most-frequently reported diseases, although stress has been identified as a risk factor for heart disease more than any other cause of death.

Survey questions about work stress in particular revealed that only 20 percent of Canadian workers felt they experienced high job strain, that is, felt they were in hectic jobs, subject to conflicting demands, and had little freedom in controlling the pace of their work or in deciding how to carry out their duties. This low percentage of job strain among workers, and the additional finding that less than 10 percent of Canadians reported dissatisfaction with their work, speaks well for the relationship between Canadians and their jobs. Nonetheless, in the small portion experiencing job strain, women were over-represented (on the other hand, job dissatisfaction was the same for men and women).

After follow-up surveys, the authors of the health report conclude that, despite their greater likelihood of experiencing stress and suffering chronic health conditions (especially the potentially fatal respiratory diseases), women received less negative impact over the long term. Perhaps more resilient, according to the authors, women were less likely to report ill health and less likely to die than men with the same conditions.

These conclusions confirm the persistent findings of many studies, especially in the U.S., that women are more likely to have chronic diseases than men, yet are less likely to die of them. Increased labour force participation has done little to change this finding. Moreover, there is little evidence that dire consequences for women will come out of this increased participation. Concerns about these consequences have placed an overemphasis on the strain aspects of work to the neglect of its rewarding aspects. Contrary to long-held beliefs, men have found work rewarding for many years. The Canadian health surveys mentioned earlier found only 17 percent of men reporting job stress. In light of the century-old assumption that men have been dying off early because of work stress, this percentage appears remarkably low.

Women have similarly found work to be rewarding. It can offer such rewards as self-esteem, recognition, prestige, and a regular pay cheque. Studies have shown that the death rates of women employed outside the home are lower than those not employed and that employed women have lower or equal prevalence of coronary heart disease.[146] Employed women also report better general health than those not employed. One extensive study involving the entire labour force of Wisconsin showed that the gap between male and female death rates did not narrow among those in the labour force compared to the general population. In fact, working men continued to experience substantially higher death rates than working women.[147] The study also explored whether working women's death rates were catching up to men's for lifestyle diseases and found that gaps were still large, especially for heart disease.

Perhaps it is not employment versus non-employment that could cause women's death rates to draw closer to men's. Instead it could be the multiple roles that women are increasingly juggling as they try to be worker, wife, and mother. Assuming that a woman has a finite amount of energy, occupying more than one role could place a serious drain on the supply and create psychological distress as she attempts to meet all her role obligations. Experts in the field of sociology and social psychology would disagree. A competing theory to limited human energy is the argument that it can expand. Women can add more roles without exhaustion because the rewards of self-esteem and other benefits of work more than offset the cost.[148]

The work role can also help in another way. It can buffer women from the stress of nonworkplace roles, especially the role of mother. High in demand and low in control, these traditional roles for women have the major elements that have been identified as villains in workplace stress. It now appears that the stress a woman experiences as a mother may be mitigated by paid work. More specifically, in a study where women self-reported role overload (having too many demands) and role conflict (having conflicting demands), only those who were not employed also reported symptoms of stress.

Stress, a risk factor for heart disease, has so far not made a dent in the longevity gap. Describing the improved health of employed married women over the past two decades, gerontologist Lois Verbrugge states that there is no indication that multiple roles are impairing women's health.[149] Epidemiologist Deborah Wingard simply points out that mortality rates from coronary heart disease have continued to decline for women despite rising employment.[150] Women's mortality rates from stomach and colon cancer (shown to be associated with stress in some studies) have also decreased dramatically in the decades since they went to work in such numbers.[151] It is true that changes in lifestyles do not show up immediately in mortality rates. Like all good medical researchers, Verbrugge suggests a need for statistical patience until the women who have made those lifestyle changes die.

CHAPTER 10

Unknowns in the New Century

What the new century will bring in matters of life and death even the World Health Organization cannot predict with certainty. We have only to look back over a hundred years for evidence that human prediction has its limits. During that period there were unforeseen developments that even the most imaginative of futurists missed as they stood on the threshold of the twentieth century.

In 1900, for example, there was every reason to believe that vaccines or other forms of immunization would soon be discovered for the major infectious diseases that took most lives. Only 15 years earlier medical science pioneers had discovered that diphtheria, which had killed thousands in worldwide epidemics in the early and middle years of the nineteenth century, was caused by a soluble toxin. With this breakthrough other scientists had gone on to find a way to neutralize the toxin's deadly effects with antitoxin they produced in immunized animals. In addition, the work of Louis Pasteur in developing a vaccine for rabies and anthrax and the discovery by Robert Koch of a test for tuberculosis were giant steps in the battle against newly-identified bacteria. In light of these discoveries the future looked bright for the control of many infectious diseases, especially diseases of childhood. Indeed, optimistic predictions proved to be accurate for diphtheria, scarlet fever, and whooping cough, which declined steadily after the discovery of antitoxins and vaccines. At the same time, continuing improvements in public health measures related to milk and water brought a striking reduction in typhoid fever.

What had not been foreseen, however, was that a whole new set of causes of death would soon challenge medical science.

Gradually freed from the risks of childhood mortality, more people in advanced countries of the world would begin to reach old age than at any previous time in history and would begin to die of diseases associated with the elderly. For these degenerative diseases, not caused by bacteria or viruses, vaccines and antitoxins and (later) antibiotics would not provide a cure. Degenerative diseases, chief among them heart disease, were not strangers to medical science at the beginning of the century; it was their growing predominance among causes of death that was new and the shift to lifestyle rather than bacterial risk factors. And there was another surprise. The degenerative diseases took a greater toll on the lives of men than women. Sadly, as the century progressed, the new gains in lifespans brought about by medical discoveries and public health measures were not evenly spread between the sexes.

There were other unpredicted developments in the twentieth century that kept men from getting the full advantage of longer lifespans. The world was becoming more urban, a trend started in the nineteenth century especially in the advanced countries, a necessary result of industrialization and the centralization of industry. But it was not urbanization itself that came as a surprise, it was the lifestyle changes that went along with it.

In recently-industrialized countries where the rosiest future seemed to revolve around greater and greater industrialization, not many would have guessed that, as the century moved along, blue-collar jobs would decrease while white-collar jobs increased resulting in a more sedentary labour force. Even the remaining blue-collar jobs required less physical activity over a shorter number of hours as automation improved. Sedentary lifestyles only added to the new risks of heart disease. So while workers in the factories of Dickens' time had been killed off by overwork and consumption, workers in the twentieth century could be killed off by lack of physical activity and heart disease.

There was another unexpected consequence of urbanization: food processing became a major industry as people looked for more convenient ways to feed their families. The consumption of fresh foods gradually dropped, especially fresh fruits and vegetables, and fast foods took their place. Higher urban incomes also led to higher consumption of meat and it would have been news to people at the beginning of the twentieth century that such a diet was anything but a boon to civilization. Realization of its effects on cholesterol levels would come later, after mid-century. By then many men in more developed countries had become big eaters—and especially big meat-eaters—and the extra pounds and extra cholesterol gave them an edge in heart disease mortality.

One of the biggest surprises of twentieth century urbanization was the way society embraced the automobile. At the beginning of the century there was no shortage of visionaries who predicted an exciting new world as a result of this invention, but not one could have predicted the dramatic cultural shift it would bring about in the more advanced countries of the world over the next hundred years. The periodical *Scientific American*, for example, predicted quieter, more relaxed cities in the new century with the demise of noisy horse-drawn vehicles:

> The improvement in city conditions by the general adoption of the motorcar can hardly be overestimated. Streets clean, dustless and odorless, with light rubber tired vehicles moving swiftly and noiselessly over their smooth expanse, would eliminate a greater part of the nervousness, distraction, and strain of modern metropolitan life.[152]

And eventually, another periodical predicted in 1904, city density problems would be solved by a mass movement of the working class to suburbia:

> Imagine a healthier race of workingmen, toiling in cheerful and sanitary factories, with mechanical skill and trade-craft developed to the highest, as the machinery grows more delicate and perfect, who, in the late afternoon, glide away in their own comfortable vehicles to their little farms or houses in the country or by the sea twenty or thirty miles distant![153]

Even by the 1920s, after the mass production of automobiles had increased car ownership in the U.S. to over 55 percent of all families (and almost a fifth of those families owned two or more cars), the great urban dream was showing signs of tarnish. In the country with the highest automobile use in the world, the construction of streets and highways was the second largest item of governmental expenditure. Social and economic historian Thomas Cochran comments: "No one has or perhaps can reliably estimate the vast size of capital invested in reshaping society to fit the automobile."[154] Automobile historian Blaine Brownell notes that the late twentieth century seeds of discontent with the automobile were already beginning to germinate in the 1920s: "... the same automobile that was supposed to decentralize the city and improve urban access to the countryside acted paradoxically to render the city even more congested."[155] There was also a rising concern about the growing toll of deaths and injuries.

Automobile traffic fatalities would continue to grow from the 1920s to the 1970s in advanced countries before they began to decline. While most of the decline is attributed to safety improvements in cars and highways and to lower speed limits, a good portion can be attributed to educational safety programs aimed at lower consumption of alcohol. Through the peak years, the message of the connection between traffic fatalities and alcohol failed to get through to drivers, especially male drivers, who outnumbered female drivers in fatal crashes while drinking by a ratio of eight to one. Who could have predicted at the beginning of the twentieth century that the much-sought after new invention would become one of the leading causes of death, surpassing the old enemy of infectious diseases after mid-century? It was as if the automobile had turned on its greatest fan, the male driver.

Today in developing countries motor vehicle fatalities have also become a leading cause of death as urbanization increases and the developing world adopts some of the risky lifestyles of the developed world. While traffic fatalities were declining in developed countries after 1970, they increased by 150 percent in Asia and 300 percent in Africa. The World Health Organization predicts that they will have tripled again on both continents by 2020. Over 750,000 people in the world now die from car crashes annually, most of them in developing countries.[156]

These were not the only surprises of urbanization in the twentieth century. The move away from rural life meant less need for large families for agricultural work. Birth rates began to drop throughout the century, a development few could have predicted, given that families of 7 to 12 children were still common at the end of the nineteenth century. Lower birth rates also led to dramatic changes for women. Fewer pregnancies and fewer child care years opened the way for them to consider employment outside the home. The time seemed right for women to act with greater independence—there had been progress, not always steady, from the first suffrage victory in Canada in 1916 to a role for women in the second World War, both in and out of the armed services, to a strong women's movement from the 1960s to the end of the century. A combination of this progress and lower childbirth mortality over a hundred years served to increase the gap that was growing between men's and women's lifespans.

The best of futurists failed to predict many of these twentieth century developments. How could they have predicted two world wars that took many young lives (many more men than women) or the sudden boom in the cigarette industry that lasted 80 years following World War I, especially when tobacco smoking had actually been around for centuries? And although the exciting possibilities for easier and faster international travel were not difficult to imagine at the turn of the century, few could have foreseen that international travellers carrying bacteria and viruses could turn localized epidemics into worldwide epidemics.

The spread of influenza in 1918 and 1919 from England and the continent to nearly every corner of the world was made easier by new technologies in transportation and the new travelling lifestyles that followed. Requirements for the vaccination of travellers improved the situation during the century but it was impossible for medical science to foresee hitherto unknown viruses and, even when they were discovered, immunization was usually not a possibility. The ease and popularity of international travel had increased a hundredfold by the late 1970s when it was discovered that an invisible passenger (the HIV virus causing AIDS) was being carried across international borders as fast as the latest jets could make the trip. While there is still controversy about its country of origin, the virus spread across North America, western Europe, Africa, Latin America, and the Caribbean within a short time; and eventually into eastern Europe, India, China, other Asian countries, and the middle east. From 26 cases of AIDS diagnosed in the U.S. in 1980 and 1981, 17 in France, and 19 in other European countries,[157] the global total became 35 million after only two decades. In developed countries, six times more men than women died of AIDS during that period; in developing countries, especially in sub-Saharan nations of Africa, the toll was spread more evenly. In Africa, with 25 million of the 35 million total cases, the epidemic of AIDS set back progress in lifespans for both sexes because of a remarkable death rate among children; in developed countries with approximately 3 million AIDS cases the setback was smaller and was primarily for men.

At the beginning of the twenty-first century we are faced with a whole new set of unknowns. With advances in technology since the beginning of the last century we can make fairly accurate projections for the next 20 years, as long as current trends hold. World Health Organization (WHO) researchers have gone that far with some confidence and some of their projections are presented here. But beyond that there is little certainty. Even a quarter-century ago it would have been difficult to envision thousands of personal computers connected with each other in homes throughout the world or the sudden appearance and spread of a deadly virus like HIV which some scientists claim may have existed as a latent human parasite for up to 100 years (and even as an animal virus for up to 200 years). We do know the world will change as a result of recent human genome discoveries, successes at cloning human embryos, and global climate changes, but how and when these changes will manifest themselves are the surprises in store for us in the twenty-first century. How they may affect the gap in male and female lifespans is an important piece of the many missing pieces. Projections for the next 20 years by WHO researchers are based on some clear assumptions: a substantial shift in the age-pattern of mortality from younger to older ages; a decline in the traditional infectious diseases although pneumonia will continue to be a leading cause of death worldwide; a substantial decline in deaths of childbirth and early infancy in the developing countries following the twentieth century pattern in developed countries; and a dramatic rise in the HIV epidemic in India, China, and east Asian countries, while rates may level off or decline in developed countries. The exception is Russia and Eastern Europe, where infection rates are currently as alarming as those of east Asia.[158] Given these scenarios, the World Health Organization projects that by 2020 cardiovascular diseases will still be the leading causes of death throughout the world. Mortality from chronic respiratory diseases such as bronchitis and emphysema will double, moving them from sixth in ranking to third, and deaths from lung cancer are also expected to double, causing it to rise from tenth to fifth place. Most of the increases in chronic respiratory diseases and lung cancer are projected to occur in developing countries, mostly among males who began smoking in large numbers in the last decades of the twentieth century. Road traffic accidents will rise from tenth to sixth place largely due to increases in developing countries where car accidents are expected to take the lives of two million people in 2020.

The ranking of AIDS among causes of death is projected to show the greatest change. Ranked 30th among causes worldwide in the 1990s, it will jump to ninth place by 2020 as HIV infections continue to climb in many developing countries. WHO projects 1.2 million HIV deaths in the world in 2020 compared to 300,000 in 1990. Of 1.2 million projected deaths, 465,000 will occur in Africa, 392,000 in India, and 182,000 in other Asian countries. In other words, three-quarters of all deaths are projected to occur in these regions alone.

As things stand at present, there is no effective vaccine for AIDS, no cure, and many question marks about drugs that are known to extend the lives of many AIDS patients. Recent findings from U.S.

tests show resistance to AIDS drugs in about half of 200,000 HIV patients tested. The author of the study, Dr. Douglas Richman of the University of California at San Diego, describes this high prevalence of drug resistance as "a bit scary." It means, according to the U.S. Center for Disease Control and Prevention, that prevention is still the most reliable route for control of AIDS.[159]

WHO projections of mortality patterns over the next twenty years also take into account the complex relationship between HIV and tuberculosis. Although mortality from tuberculosis fell throughout the twentieth century as a result of vaccination, early detection, and drug therapy, it has emerged as a frequent opportunistic infection occurring in AIDS patients, especially in Africa and Haiti. And as with the HIV virus, new forms of mycobacteria causing AIDS-related tuberculosis appear to be resistant to drugs.

These projections for specific causes of death lay the groundwork for WHO projections for life expectancy. Life expectancy at birth is projected to increase in all regions. In many developed countries life expectancy for females may reach 88. Smaller gains are projected across the world for males as compared with females, smaller gains that are in large part due to the greater impact of the tobacco epidemic on males. In actual years, women in developed countries will gain seven compared to a gain of five for men. Even larger female gains are expected in developing countries of Africa, India, and east Asia.[160] The gap between male and female life expectancies, therefore, will continue to widen for another 20 years if WHO projections become reality.

Besides the basic assumptions underlying WHO projections, there are many other variables that could affect world mortality rates in the twenty-first century. And if and when they do make themselves felt, their impact is far from clear. The exciting progress in human genome discoveries is one such area. There are many unknowns in the relationship between DNA and genes and the proteins they are associated with, but the study of genes is going ahead so rapidly that the total story will soon be known and the diagnosis and treatment of disease in the twenty-first century will be forever changed.

The female advantage of two X chromosomes and the resulting mosaic nature of female cells described in chapter 2 have made a contribution to longer lives for women. The size of the contribution has been unknown in the past; it may become more clearly defined as new findings indicate which of the body's proteins and their functions are connected with which gene (or combination of genes) located on the chromosomes. More important in trying to envision future longevity gaps between men and women will be discoveries of genes connected with specific diseases that are now known to take more male than female lives.

If advance knowledge about our gene make-up allows each individual a glimpse of his or her potential future health, it is anybody's guess what we will do with that knowledge. We might adopt preventive lifestyles or we might leave the outcome completely in the hands of scientists who, armed with new genetic knowledge, will soon provide cures. A whole new set of personal decisions, therefore, may face us when the next phase of the genome age is completed. And to complicate matters further, we have no way of knowing this early in the century what sanctions imposed by health care systems throughout the world might help us make up our minds.

If genome discoveries have created tensions between public and private scientific interests, they will pale in comparison to what will take place over the next few decades in the area of human cloning. When the dust settles following the controversy—when national governments sort out the ethical issues and find a way for scientists (predominantly private sector scientists at present) to use cloned embryos to cure diseases without producing new human life—there will be new issues as yet unforeseen as researchers begin to replace damaged human cells with undamaged cloned cells. And it is almost certain that some diseases will benefit more than others. Most frequently mentioned by researchers are diabetes and neurodegenerative disorders such as Parkinson's and Alzheimer disease and, less frequently, stroke and cancer. Since all these causes of death affect men more than women—especially diabetes and cancer where the mortality ratio is 1.5 to one—there could be some changes to male life expectancy vis-à-vis female life expectancy before the century is out.

Global climate change may also affect human health in the twenty-first century. Because of greenhouse gas emissions, global temperatures have risen over the past quarter century and climatologists predict the trend will continue. The gradual and complex nature of the changes makes it difficult to predict the environmental consequences. WHO studies indicate that an average global temperature increase of even one to two degrees Celsius would extend the range of mosquitos in Asia and Africa to new areas of higher altitude, leading to increases in cases of malaria. Present annual deaths of two to three million could rise to five million. If global warming also increases rainfall, local flooding could allow even greater levels of mosquito breeding. Such changes, of course, would affect life expectancies only in Africa and some Asian countries including India, but with 15 percent more male than female deaths from malaria annually the changes are likely to widen the male-female life expectancy gap in those parts of the developing world.

In addition, continued rising trends in greenhouse gas emissions could increase risks of cardiovascular and respiratory illnesses. These diseases are especially vulnerable to the effects of atmospheric particulate matter produced by the burning of fossil fuels. The World Health Organization predicts that 700,000 additional deaths could occur annually because of the additional exposure. And if current mortality trends continue, men will be twice as likely as women to be included in these 700,000 deaths.

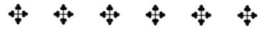

With varying stages of social and economic development across the world, the gains in lifespan for men will be uneven in the first part of the twenty-first century, but in general men will continue to die before women. The growing predominance of degenerative diseases means lifestyle behaviours like smoking, drinking, and overeating will continue to make the largest contribution to the male-female difference. These behaviours are simply a matter of taking known risks and can be added to the risks associated with motor vehicle fatalities that tend to take the lives of men long before they grow old.

In this scenario for the future, health policymakers (and women) need to understand better the motivation behind risk-taking by men. Assuming that men know the health risks very well, there are a few possible reasons for their willingness to take them. Either they underestimate the effect of these risks on themselves individually ("poor health outcomes may happen to others, but they won't happen to me"), or long life is not a cherished goal, not an attractive prospect despite a growing list of active older men like economist and writer John Galbraith, 94, government adviser Mitchell Sharp, 91, actor Gregory Peck, 86, and television commentator Mike Wallace, 84. Or perhaps men have nothing against long life but value it less than personal independence and the ability to control their own destinies.

Whatever the motivation of men, women would do well to take their own destinies in hand and consider marrying men four to six years younger than themselves.

Endnotes

[1] Lois M. Verbrugge, The twain meet: Empirical explanations of sex differences in health and mortality (an analysis of data from the Health in Detroit Study, a survey of 714 adults in the Detroit metropolitan area), in *Gender, Health, and Longevity, Multidisciplinary Perspectives*, M.G. Ory and H.R. Warner, eds., 1990.

[2] Verbrugge, Gender and health: An update on hypotheses and evidence, *Journal of Health and Social Behavior*, 1985; Kenneth G. Manton, Population models of gender differences in mortality, morbidity and disability risks, in *Gender, Health, and Longevity, Multidisciplinary Perspectives*, 1990; Deborah L. Wingard, The sex differential: Morbidity, mortality, and lifestyle, *American Review of Public Health*, 1984.

[3] The *United Nations Statistical Year Book 1996* gives the following low infant mortality rates: Japan, 4 per 1,000 births; Finland, 5; Iceland, 5; Norway, 5; Singapore, 5; Sweden, 5; Switzerland, 5; Sweden, 5; Canada, 6; Hong Kong, 6.

[4] Gy. Acsádi and J. Nemeskéri, *History of Human Lifespan and Mortality*, 1970, p. 86.

[5] Statistics Canada, *Age-standardized mortality rates*, 1997.

[6] R. Pressat, Surmortalité biologique et surmortalité sociale, *Revue française sociologie*, 1973.

[7] Lois M. Verbrugge, Gender and health: An update on hypotheses and evidence, 1985.

[8] Ingrid Waldron, Sex differences in human mortality: The role of genetic factors, *Social Science and Medicine*, 1983.

[9] David W.E. Smith, *Human Longevity*, 1993, p. 90.

[10] Tessa M. Pollard, Sex, gender and cardiovascular disease, in *Sex, Gender and Health*, Tessa M. Pollard and S.B. Hyatt, eds., 1999.

[11] William R. Hazzard, A central role of sex hormones in the sex differential in lipoprotein metabolism, atherosclerosis, and longevity, in *Gender, Health, and Longevity, Multidisciplinary Perspectives*, Ory and Warner, eds., 1990.

[12] There is a downside to the female tendency to produce more antibodies. As they grow older women also produce more autoantibodies, that is, they produce more antibodies that fight substances that are naturally present in the body rather than foreign substances that are not welcome. As a result, women are more inclined to develop autoimmune diseases like rheumatoid arthritis, lupus, and myasthenia gravis.

[13] Marc E. Weksler, A possible role for the immune system in the gender-longevity differential, in *Gender, Health, and Longevity, Multidisciplinary Perspectives*, 1990.

[14] F.J. Grundbacher, Human X chromosome carries quantitative genes for immunoglobulin M, *Science*, 1972.

[15] Ingrid Waldron, What do we know about causes of sex differences in mortality? A review of the literature, *Population Bulletin of the United Nations*, 1985.

[16] Constance Holden, Why do women live longer than men? *Science*, 1987.

[17] David W.E. Smith and H.R. Warner, Overview of biomedical perspectives: Possible relations between genes on the sex chromosomes and longevity, in *Gender, Health, and Longevity, Multdisciplinary Perspectives*, 1990.

[18] Tessa Pollard, Sex, gender and cardiovascular disease.

[19] Tessa Pollard.

[20] Catherine M. Stoney et al., Sex differences in physiological responses to stress and in coronary heart disease: A causal link? *Psychophysiology*, 1987.

[21] Heino F.L. Meyer-Bahlburg, Aggression, androgens, and the XYY syndrome, in *Sex Differences in Behavior*, R.C. Friedman et al., eds., 1974.

[22] Heino Meyer-Bahlburg.

[23] K. Rhodes et al., Immunoglobulins and the X chromosome, *British Medical Journal*, 1969.

[24] United Nations Secretariat, *World Health Statistics Annual 1995*.

[25] Statistics Canada, Health Statistics Division, *Selected Leading Causes of Death*, 1997.

[26] United Nations Secretariat, Sex differentials in life expectancy and mortality in developed countries: An analysis by age groups and causes of death from recent and historical data, *Population Bulletin of the United Nations*, 1988.

[27] David S. Krantz et al., Environmental stress and biobehavioral antecedents of coronary heart disease, *Journal of Consulting and Clinical Psychology*, 1988.

[28] L.H. Epstein and K.A. Perkins, Smoking, stress, and coronary heart disease, *Journal of Consulting and Clinical Psychology*, 1988.

[29] United Nations Secretariat, *Population Newsletter*, 1997.

[30] Statistics Canada, Health Statistics Division, *Report on Smoking Prevalence in Canada, 1985 to 1999*, January 2000.

[31] Valentin Fuster et al., Platelet survival and the development of coronary artery disease in the young adult: Effects of cigarette smoking, strong family history and medical therapy, *Circulation*, 1981.

[32] Carl G. Becker and Theodore Dubin, Activation of factor XII by tobacco glycoprotein, *Journal of Experimental Medicine*, 1977.

[33] Susan S. Girdler, et al., Smoking status and nicotine administration differentially modify hemodynamic stress reactivity in men and women, *Psychosomatic Medicine*, 1997.

[34] Peter H. Levine, An acute effect of cigarette smoking on platelet function, *Circulation*, 1973.

[35] R.D. Retherford, *The Changing Sex Differential in Mortality*, 1975.

[36] David W.E. Smith, *Human Longevity*, 1993.

[37] David S. Krantz et al.

[38] Organization for Economic Cooperation and Development, *Labour Force Statistics 1978-1998*, Paris, 1999.

[39] C.A. Nathanson, Sex differences in mortality, *Annual Review of Sociology*, 1984.

[40] Leonard H. Epstein and Kenneth A. Perkins.

[41] Statistics Canada, *National Population Health Survey 1996-97*, Ottawa, 1998.

[42] *National Population Health Survey 1996-97.*

[43] *National Population Health Survey 1996-97.*

[44] Statistics Canada, *Health Improvement Measures*, 1997. Of those who reported they were taking measures, 30 percent of women and 28 percent of men were increasing their level of exercise; 6.5 percent of women and 4.5 percent of men were losing weight; 6 percent of women and 4 percent of men were improving their eating habits; and 2.5 percent of women and less than one percent of men were drinking less alcohol. Two and a half percent of both men and women reported they were quitting or reducing smoking.

[45] Statistics Canada, *The Changing Face of Heart Disease and Stroke in Canada 2000*, October 1999.

[46] Quoted in Vilhjalmur Stefansson, *Cancer: Disease of Civilization?* 1960, p. 37.

[47] Stefansson, p. 56.

[48] Statistics Canada, *Historical Statistics*, 1983. Comparisons across the century are difficult. The system of classification of deaths by cause changes from time to time to be consistent with current medical knowledge and terminology.

[49] Canada, Dominion Bureau of Statistics, *Health Reference Book 1946*, 1947.

[50] Canada, Dominion Bureau of Statistics, *Special Report on Contributory Causes of Death 1926*, 1929.

[51] United Nations, *World Health Statistics Annual*, 1995.

[52] Vincent T. DeVita, Jr. et al., eds., *Cancer, Principles and Practice of Oncology*, 2001.

[53] National Cancer Institute of Canada, *Canadian Cancer Statistics*, 2000.

[54] Canadian Cancer Society, *Facts on Lung Cancer*, 2000.

[55] Statistics Canada, *Report on Smoking Prevalence in Canada 1985 to 1999*, January, 2000.

[56] M.C. Pike, Epidemiology of cancer, in *Introduction to the Cellular and Molecular Biology of Cancer*, L.M. Franks and N. Teich, eds.

[57] Paul C. Weiler, *Protecting the Worker from Disability: Challenges for the Eighties*, 1983, p. 26.

[58] Annalee Yassi, *Occupational Disease and Workers' Compensation in Ontario*, 1983, p. 125-126.

[59] *Introduction to the Cellular and Molecular Biology of Cancer*, p. 89.

[60] Barbara A. Plog et al., *Fundamentals of Industrial Hygiene*, 1996, p. 134.

[61] Sandra M. Levy, *Behavior and Cancer*, 1985, p. 43.

[62] R. Doll and R. Peto, *The Causes of Cancer: Quantitative Estimates of Avoidable Risks of Cancer in the United States Today*, 1981.

[63] M.C. Pike, Epidemiology of cancer.

[64] Sandra M. Levy, *Behavior and Cancer*, p. 34.

[65] National Cancer Institute, *Canadian Cancer Statistics*, p. 13.

[66] Statistics Canada, *National Population Health Survey 1996-97.*

[67] Statistics Canada, Alcohol use and its consequences, *Canadian Social Trends*, 1995.

[68] Sandra M. Levy, *Behavior and Cancer*, p. 71. This evidence was consistent in both

epidemiological and laboratory studies.

[69] Barry Halliwell and J.M.C. Gutteridge, *Free Radicals in Biology and Medicine*, 1985. Oversimplifying perhaps, a free radical is an unpaired electron that has been pulled away from a molecule during a chemical reaction. Its damage is done when it absorbs other electrons from normal body cells in trying to make a new pair. The process of damage by oxygen radicals, called oxidation, is slowed down or prevented by anti-oxidants found naturally in the body (often enzymes and other compounds) and by anti-oxidants obtained from diet.

[70] The red in tomatoes lowers risk of disease, researchers discover, *Winnipeg Free Press*, November 5, 1997, p. D4.

[71] Statistics Canada, *Vital Statistics Compendium 1996*.

[72] National Cancer Institute of Canada, *Canadian Cancer Statistics 2000*.

[73] Body mass index is calculated by dividing weight in kilograms by the square of height in metres.

[74] Statistics Canada, *Health Reports*, 2001.

[75] United Nations, Symposium on health and mortality, *Population Newsletter*, 1997.

[76] World Health Organization, *Summary: The Global Burden of Disease*, C.J.L. Murray and A.D. Lopez, eds., 1996.

[77] WHO, *Summary: The Global Burden of Disease*.

[78] Editorial, Tobacco's toll, *Lancet*, 1992.

[79] Descriptions of the workings of the respiratory system used here are a condensed version of descriptions given in the *Johns Hopkins Medical Handbook*, ed., Simeon Margolis, 1995.

[80] E.M. Makomaski Illing and M.J. Kaiserman, Mortality attributable to tobacco use in Canada and its regions, 1994 and 1996, *Chronic Diseases in Canada*, 1999.

[81] W.H.H. Andrews, *Liver*, 1979.

[82] World Health Organization, *The Global Burden of Disease*, 1996.

[83] Statistics Canada, Alcohol use and its consequences, *Canadian Social Trends*, 1995.

[84] Editorial, Theories of addiction, *Addiction*, 2001.

[85] J. Benjamin et al., Population and familial association between the D4 dopamine receptor gene and measures of novelty seeking, *Nature Genetics*, 1996.

[86] R.W. Jeffery, Risk behavior and health, *American Psychologist*, 1989.

[87] R.W. Jeffery, Risk behavior and health.

[88] R.W. Jeffery, Risk behavior and health.

[89] J. Frank Yates, *Risk-Taking Behavior*, 1991, p. 233.

[90] K. Deaux, From individual differences to social categories, *American Psychologist*, 1984.

[91] D.N. Ruble and T.L. Ruble, Sex stereotypes, in *In the Eye of the Beholder, Contemporary Issues in Stereotyping,* ed. Arthur G. Miller, 1982.

[92] C. McCauley et al., Stereotyping: From prejudice to prediction, *Psychological Bulletin*, 1980.

[93] Ruble and Ruble, 1982.

94 *Population Bulletin of the United Nations*, 1985.

95 Statistics Canada, *Mortality: Summary List of Causes*, 1995.

96 Statistics Canada, *Health Reports 1995*, p. 12.

97 Statistics Canada, Accidents in Canada, 1988 and 1993, *Health Reports 1995*. Over 65 years of age, women have a higher rate of non-fatal accidents.

98 Statistics Canada, *Vital Statistics Compendium 1996*, 1999. Accidental falls are the next major cause, making up 31 percent of total accident fatalities, excluding suicide and homicide deaths. Falls are the leading cause of accidental death among the elderly.

99 Alcohol use and its consequences, *Canadian Social Trends*, autumn 1995.

100 Transport Canada, *Alcohol Use Among Persons Fatally Injured in Motor Vehicle Accidents: Canada*, 1991.

101 Alcohol use and its consequences.

102 Alcohol use and its consequences.

103 A.F. Williams and A.K. Lund, Seat belt use laws and occupant crash protection in the United States, *American Journal of Public Health*, 1986. Enforcement of seat belt laws is also an important variable. Canada has been credited with a greater level of enforcement than that of the U.S., resulting in rates of over 60 percent in the 1980s. By the year 2000 seat belt usage in Canada reached over 90 percent.

104 Statistics Canada, *Selected Leading Causes of Death*, 1997.

105 Canada, *Suicide in Canada, Report of the National Task Force on Suicide in Canada*, 1987.

106 World Health Organization, *Summary: The Global Burden of Disease*, C.J.L. Murray and A.D. Lopez, eds., 1996.

107 John Adams, *Risk*, 1995.

108 John Adams, *Risk*, 1995.

109 M.S. Stroebe and W. Stroebe, Who suffers more? Sex differences in health risks of the widowed, *Psychological Bulletin*, 1983.

110 Debra Umberson, Family status and health behaviors: social control as a dimension of social integration, *Journal of Health and Social Behavior*, 1987.

111 Sally Wyke and Graeme Ford, Competing explanations for associations between marital status and health, *Social Science and Medicine*, 1992.

112 This is basically the thrust of the classic work of Emile Durkheim on the subject of suicide, written at the end of the nineteenth century. Twentieth century researchers have theorized that social integration, besides providing an immunity to suicide, also provides immunity to mortality more generally.

113 L.A. Lillard and C.W.A. Panis, Marital status and mortality: the role of health, *Demography*, 1996.

114 For example Bernard (1972), Gove (1973), and Kobrin and Hendershot (1977).

115 Ingrid Waldron, What do we know about causes of sex differences in mortality? A review of the literature, *Population Bulletin of the United Nations*, 1985.

116 S.M. McKinlay et al., Multiple roles for middle-aged women and their impact on health, in *Gender, Health, and Longevity, Multidisciplinary Perspectives*, Ory and Warner, eds., 1990.

[117] M.S. Stroebe and W. Stroebe, Who suffers more? Sex differences in health risks of the widowed.

[118] Debra Umberson, Family status and health behaviors: social control as a dimension of social integration.

[119] G. Pappas et al., The increasing disparity in mortality between socioeconomic groups in the United States, 1960 and 1986, *New England Journal of Medicine*, 1993.

[120] G.A. Kaplan et al., Inequality in income and mortality in the United States: analysis of mortality and potential pathways, *British Medical Journal*, 1996.

[121] Statistics Canada, Income inequality and mortality among working-age people in Canada and the US, *Health Reports*, 1999.

[122] R.G. Wilkinson, Income distribution and life expectancy, *British Medical Journal*, 1992.

[123] R.G. Wilkinson, Income and mortality, in *Class and Health*, R.G. Wilkinson, ed., 1986.

[124] World Health Organization, Social and economic differentials in mortality in developed countries, in *World Population Trends and Policies*, 1987 Monitoring Report.

[125] D.T. Wigle and Y. Mao, *Mortality by Income Level in Urban Canada*, 1980; R. Wilkins et al., Change in Mortality by Income in Urban Canada 1971-1986, *Health Reports 1989*.

[126] For example, J.P. Courteau, *Mortality among the James Bay Cree of northern Quebec: 1982-86*; Y. Mao et al., Mortality on Canadian Indian reserves 1977-1982, *Canadian Journal of Public Health*, 1986; G.K. Jarvis and M. Boldt, Death styles among Canadian Indians, *Social Science and Medicine*, 1982.

[127] G.A. Kaplan et al., Inequality in income and mortality in the United States: analysis of mortality and potential pathways.

[128] T. Hirayama, quoted in Simon P. Thomas and Steve E. Hrudey, *Risk of Death in Canada, What We Know and How We Know It*, 1997.

[129] R.G. Wilkinson, Income distribution and life expectancy.

[130] R.G. Wilkinson, Income and mortality.

[131] W.J. Millar, Sex differentials in mortality by income level in urban Canada, *Canadian Journal of Public Health*, 1983.

[132] K.R. Smith and N.J. Waitzman, Double jeopardy: interaction effects of marital and poverty status on the risk of mortality, *Demography*, 1994.

[133] James S. House et al., Excess mortality among urban residents: how much, for whom, and why? *American Journal of Public Health*, 2000.

[134] Kathryn Wilkins, Causes of death: How the sexes differ, *Health Reports*, Statistics Canada, 1995.

[135] *The Global Burden of Disease Vol. 1*, C.J.L. Murray and Alan D. Lopez, eds., World Health Organization, 1996.

[136] UN Secretariat, Symposium on health and mortality, *Population Newsletter*, 1997.

[137] *United Nations Statistical Yearbook*, 1996.

[138] *Population Bulletin of the United Nations*, 1988, using data from the early 1980s.

[139] S.H. Preston, *Mortality Patterns in National Populations*, 1976.

[140] Simon P. Thomas and Steve E. Hrudey, *Risk of Death in Canada, What We Know and*

How We Know It, 1997.

[141] Richard Peto et al., Mortality from tobacco in developed countries: indirect estimation from national vital statistics, *Lancet*, 1992.

[142] E.M.M. Illing and M.J. Kaiserman, Mortality attributable to tobacco use in Canada and its regions, 1994 and 1996, *Chronic Diseases in Canada*, 1999.

[143] In the U.S., for example, per capita alcohol consumption dropped 17 percent between 1977 and 1998. See Apparent per capita ethanol consumption for the United States, *Alcohol Epidemiologic Data System*, 1998. Government reports also show a decrease of 25 percent over the same period in total alcohol-related mortality.

[144] Lois Verbrugge, Gender and health: An update on hypotheses and evidence, *Journal of Health and Social Behavior*, 1985.

[145] Statistics Canada, *Health Report*, 2001. This question was one of five parts of a measure of stress that included trying to take on too much at once, feeling pressure to be like other people, feeling that others expect too much, feeling that your work around the home is not appreciated, and feeling that others are too critical of you.

[146] Deborah Wingard, The sex differential in morbidity, mortality, and lifestyle, *Annual Review of Public Health*, 1984; M.R.C. Passannante and C. Nathanson, Women in the labor force: Are sex mortality differentials changing? *Journal of Occupational Medicine*, 1987; David Krantz et al., Environmental stress and biobehavioral antecedents of coronary heart disease, *Journal of Consulting and Clinical Psychology*, 1988; C.D. Zick and K.R. Smith, Marital transitions, poverty, and gender differences in mortality, *Journal of Marriage and the Family*, 1991.

[147] M.R.C. Passannante and C. Nathanson, Women in the labor force: Are sex mortality differentials changing?

[148] Rosalind Barnett, Multiple roles, gender, and psychological distress, in *Handbook of Stress, Theoretical and Clinical Aspects*, eds. L. Goldberger and S. Breznitz, 1993.

[149] Lois Verbrugge, Gender and health: An update on hypotheses and evidence.

[150] Deborah Wingard, The sex differential in morbidity, mortality, and lifestyle.

[151] National Cancer Institute of Canada, *Canadian Cancer Statistics 2000*.

[152] James J. Flink, *The Car Culture*, 1975, p. 39.

[153] *The Car Culture*, p. 39.

[154] *The Car Culture*, p. 141.

[155] *The Car Culture*, p. 154.

[156] Anthony J. McMichael, The urban environment and health in a world of increasing globalization: Issues for developing countries, *Bulletin of the World Health Organization*, 2001.

[157] Mirko D. Gmek, *History of AIDS, Emergence and Origin of a Modern Pandemic*, 1990.

[158] C.J.L. Murray and A.D. Lopez, *Global Burden of Disease*, 1996.

[159] Daniel Q. Haney, Virus resistance to HIV drugs grows, *Ottawa Citizen*, December 23, 2001.

[160] *Global Burden of Disease*.

Selected Bibliography

Apparent per capita ethanol consumption for the United States, *Alcohol Epidemiologic Data System*, 1998.

Acsádi, Gy and J. Nemeskéri, *History of Human Lifespan and Mortality*, Budapest: Akadémiai Kiado, 1970.

Adams, John, *Risk*, London: UCL Press, 1995.

Ames, Bruce N., Dietary carcinogens and anticarcinogens, *Science*, vol. 221, 1983.

Andrews, W.H.H., *Liver*, London: Arnold, 1979.

Barnett, Rosalind, Multiple roles, gender, and psychological distress, in *Handbook of Stress, Theoretical and Clinical Aspects*, L. Goldberger and S. Breznitz, eds., New York: Free Press, 1993.

Becker, Carl G. and Theodore Dubin, Activation of factor XII by tobacco glycoprotein, *Journal of Experimental Medicine*, vol. 146, 1977.

Bernard, Jessie, *The Future of Marriage*, New York: World Publishing, 1972.

Brancker, Anna, Lung cancer and smoking prevalence in Canada, *Health Reports*, Statistics Canada, 1990.

Canada, Dominion Bureau of Statistics, *Health Reference Book 1946*, 1947.

Canada, Dominion Bureau of Statistics, *Special Report on Contributory Causes of Death 1926*, 1929.

Canada, *Suicide in Canada, Report of the National Task Force on Suicide in Canada*, 1987.

Canadian Cancer Society, *Facts on Lung Cancer*, 2000.

Canadian Liver Foundation, *Alcohol and the Liver*, 2001.

Courteau, J.P., *Mortality among the James Bay Cree of northern Quebec: 1982-86*, Montreal: Montreal General Hospital, 1989.

Deaux, K., From individual differences to social categories, *American Psychologist*, vol. 39, no. 2, 1984.

DeVita, Jr., Vincent T. et al., eds., *Cancer, Principles and Practice of Oncology*, Philadelphia: Lippincott, Williams and Wilkins, 2001.

Doll R. and R. Peto, The causes of cancer: Quantitative estimates of avoidable risks of cancer in the United States today, *Journal of National Cancer Institute*, vol. 66, 1981.

Editorial, Tobacco's toll, *Lancet*, 1992.

Epstein, L.H. and K.A. Perkins, Smoking, stress, and coronary heart disease, *Journal of Consulting and Clinical Psychology*, vol. 56, no. 3, 1988.

Flink, James J., *The Car Culture*, Cambridge: MIT Press, 1975.

Franks, L.M. and N. Teich, eds., *Introduction to the Cellular and Molecular Biology of Cancer*, New York: Oxford University Press, 1986.

Fuster, Valentin et al., Platelet survival and the development of coronary artery disease in the young adult: Effects of cigarette smoking, strong family history and medical therapy, *Circulation*, vol. 63, no. 3, 1981.

Girdler, Susan S. et al., Smoking status and nicotine administration differentially modify hemodynamic stress reactivity in men and women, *Psychosomatic Medicine*, vol. 59, 1997.

Gmek, Mirko D., *History of AIDS, Emergence and Origin of a Modern Pandemic*, Princeton: Princeton University, 1990.

Gove, Walter R., The relationship between sex role, marital role, and mental illness, *Social Forces*, vol. 51, 1972.

Griffin, Beverly, Structure of DNA and its relationship to carcinogenesis, in *Introduction to the Cellular and Molecular Biology of Cancer*, L.M. Franks and N. Teich, eds., 1986

Grundbacher, F.J., Human X chromosome carries quantitative genes for immunoglobulin M, *Science*, vol. 176, 1972.

Halliwell, Barry and J.M.C. Gutteridge, *Free Radicals in Biology and Medicine*, Oxford: Clarendon Press, 1985.

Haney, Daniel Q., Virus resistance to HIV drugs grows, *Ottawa Citizen*, December 23, 2001.

Hazzard, William R., A central role of sex hormones in the sex differential in lipoprotein metabolism, atherosclerosis, and longevity, in *Gender, Health, and Longevity, Multidisciplinary Perspectives*, Marcia G. Ory and H.R. Warner, eds., New York: Springer Publishing, 1990.

Heart and Stroke Foundation of Canada, *Heart Disease and Stroke in Canada 1997*, Ottawa, 1997.

Hirdes, John P. and W.F. Forbes, The importance of social relationships, socioeconomic status and health practices with respect to mortality among healthy Ontario males, *Journal of Clinical Epidemiology*, vol. 45, no. 2, 1992.

Holden, Constance, Why do women live longer than men? *Science*, vol. 238, 1987.

Holliday, Robin, X chromosome reactivation, *Nature*, vol. 327, 1987.

House, James S. et al., Excess mortality among urban residents: how much, for whom, and why? *American Journal of Public Health*, vol. 90, no. 12, 2000.

Illing, E.M.M. and M.J. Kaiserman, Mortality attributable to tobacco use in Canada and its regions, 1994 and 1996, *Chronic Diseases in Canada*, vol. 20, no. 3, 1999.

Jarvis, G.K. and M. Boldt, Death styles among Canadian Indians, *Social Science and Medicine*, vol. 16, 1982.

Jeffery, R.W., Risk behavior and health, *American Psychologist*, vol. 44, no. 9, 1989.

Johns Hopkins Medical Handbook, ed., Simeon Margolis, 1995.

Kaplan, G.A. et al., Inequality in income and mortality in the United States: analysis of mortality and potential pathways, *British Medical Journal*, vol. 312, 1996.

Kobrin, Frances and G.E. Hendershot, Do family ties reduce mortality? Evidence from the United States, 1966-1968, *Journal of Marriage and the Family*, vol. 39, 1977.

Krantz, David S. et al. Environmental stress and biobehavioral antecedents of coronary heart disease, *Journal of Consulting and Clinical Psychology*, vol. 56, no. 3, 1988.

Levine, Peter H., An acute effect of cigarette smoking on platelet function, *Circulation*, vol. 48, 1973.

Levy, Sandra M., *Behavior and Cancer*, San Francisco: Jossey-Bass Publishers, 1985.

Lillard, L.A. and C.W.A. Panis, Marital status and mortality: the role of health, *Demography*, vol. 33, 1996.

Manton, Kenneth G., Population models of gender differences in mortality, morbidity and disability risks, in *Gender, Health, and Longevity, Multidisciplinary Perspectives*, Marcia G. Ory and H.R. Warner, eds., New York: Springer Publishing, 1990.

Mark, Elen and K. Wilkins, Death due to accidents, poisoning and violence among Canada's elderly: Trends from 1926 to 1985, *Chronic Diseases in Canada*, vol. 10, no. 1, 1989.

Mao, Y. et al., Mortality on Canadian Indian reserves 1977-1982, *Canadian Journal of Public Health*, vol. 77, no. 4, 1986.

McCauley, C. et al., Stereotyping: From prejudice to prediction, *Psychological Bulletin*, vol. 87, no. 1, 1980.

McKinlay, S.M. et al., Multiple roles for middle-aged women and their impact on health, in *Gender, Health and Longevity*, Marcia G. Ory and H.R. Warner, eds., New York: Springer Publishing, 1990.

McMichael, Anthony J., The urban environment and health in a world of increasing globalization: Issues for developing countries, *Bulletin of the World Health Organization*, 2001.

Meyer-Bahlburg, Heino F.L., Aggression, androgens, and the XYY syndrome, in *Sex Differences in Behavior*, Friedman R.C. et al., eds., New York: John Wiley and Sons, 1974.

Millar, W.J. Accidents in Canada, 1988 and 1993, *Health Reports 1995*, vol. 7, no. 2, Statistics Canada, 1995.

Millar, W.J. Sex differentials in mortality by income level in urban Canada, *Canadian Journal of Public Health*, vol. 74, 1983.

Nathanson, C.A., Sex differences in mortality, *Annual Review of Sociology*, vol. 10, 1984.

National Cancer Institute of Canada, *Canadian Cancer Statistics*, Toronto, 2000.

Organization for Economic Cooperation and Development, *Labour Force Statistics 1978-1998*, Paris, 1999.

Pappas, G. et al., The increasing disparity in mortality between socioeconomic groups in the United States, 1960 and 1986, *New England Journal of Medicine*, vol. 329, no. 2, 1993.

Passannante, M.R.C. and C. Nathanson, Women in the labor force: Are sex mortality differentials changing? *Journal of Occupational Medicine*, vol. 29, 1987.

Peto, Richard et al., Mortality from tobacco in developed countries: indirect estimation from national vital statistics, *Lancet*, vol. 339, 1992.

Pike, M.C., Epidemiology of cancer, in *Introduction to the Cellular and Molecular Biology of Cancer*, L.M. Franks and N. Teich, eds., New York: Oxford University Press, 1986.

Plog, Barbara A. et al., *Fundamentals of Industrial Hygiene*, National Safety Council, Itasca, Illinois, 1996.

Pollard, Tessa M., Sex, gender and cardiovascular disease, in *Sex, Gender and Health*, Tessa

M. Pollard and S.B. Hyatt, eds., Cambridge: Cambridge University Press, 1999.

Population Bulletin of the United Nations, 1985.

Population Bulletin of the United Nations, 1988.

Pressat, R., Surmortalité biologique et surmortalité sociale, *Revue francáaise sociologie*, vol. 14, 1973.

Preston, S.H., *Mortality Patterns in National Populations*, New York: Academic Press, 1976.

The red in tomatoes lowers risk of disease, researchers discover, *Winnipeg Free Press*, November 5, 1997.

Retherford, R.D., *The Changing Sex Differential in Mortality*, Westport: Greenwood Press, 1975.

Rhodes, K. et al., Immunoglobulins and the X chromosome, *British Medical Journal*, vol. 3, 1969.

Ruble, D.N. and T.L. Ruble, Sex stereotypes, in *In the Eye of the Beholder, Contemporary Issues in Stereotyping*, Arthur G. Miller, ed., New York: Praeger Scientific, 1982.

Selye, Hans, History of the stress concept, in *Handbook of Stress, Theoretical Aspects*, Leo Goldberger and Shlomo Breznitz, New York: Free Press, 1993.

Shugar, Stephen, *Effects of Asbestos in the Canadian Environment*, National Research Council, Ottawa, 1979.

Smith, David W.E., *Human Longevity*, New York: Oxford University Press, 1993.

Smith, David W.E. and H.R. Warner, Overview of biomedical perspectives: Possible relations between genes on the sex chromosomes and longevity, in *Gender, Health, and Longevity, Multidisciplinary Perspectives*, Marcia G. Ory and H.R. Warner, eds., New York: Springer Publishing, 1990.

Smith, K.R. and N.J. Waitzman, Double jeopardy: interaction effects of marital and poverty status on the risk of mortality, *Demography*, vol. 31, no. 3, 1994.

Statistics Canada, *Age-standardized mortality rates*, 1997.

Statistics Canada, Alcohol Use and its Consequences, *Canadian Social Trends*, 1995.

Statistics Canada, *The Changing Face of Heart Disease and Stroke in Canada 2000*, October 1999.

Statistics Canada, *Health Improvement Measures*, 1997.

Statistics Canada, How healthy are Canadians? *Health Reports*, vol. 12, no. 3, 2001.

Statistics Canada, *Historical Statistics*, 1983.

Statistics Canada, Income inequality and mortality among working-age people in Canada and the US, *Health Reports*, vol. 11, no. 3, 1999.

Statistics Canada, *Mortality: Summary List of Causes*, 1995.

Statistics Canada, *National Population Health Survey 1996-97*, Ottawa, 1998.

Statistics Canada, *Report on Smoking Prevalence in Canada 1985 to 1999*, January, 2000.

Statistics Canada, *Selected Leading Causes of Death*, 1997.

Statistics Canada, *Vital Statistics Compendium 1996*, Ottawa, 1999.

Stefansson, Vilhjalmur, *Cancer: Disease of Civilization?* New York: Hill and Wang, 1960.

Stoney, Catherine M. et al., Sex differences in physiological responses to stress and in coronary heart disease: A causal link? *Psychophysiology,* vol. 24, no. 2, 1987.

Stroebe, M.S. and W. Stroebe, Who suffers more? Sex differences in health risks of the widowed, *Psychological Bulletin,* vol. 93, no. 2, 1983.

Thomas, Simon P. and Steve E. Hrudey, *Risk of Death in Canada, What We Know and How We Know It,* Edmonton: University of Alberta, 1997.

Transport Canada, *Alcohol Use Among Persons Fatally Injured in Motor Vehicle Accidents: Canada,* 1991.

Umberson, Debra, Family status and health behaviors: social control as a dimension of social integration, *Journal of Health and Social Behavior,* vol. 28, 1987.

United Nations Secretariat, World population monitoring, 1998: Health and mortality, *Population Newsletter,* 1997.

United Nations Secretariat, Sex differentials in life expectancy and mortality in developed countries: An analysis by age groups and causes of death from recent and historical data, *Population Bulletin of the United Nations,* no. 25, 1988.

United Nations Secretariat, Sex differentials in survivorship in the developing world: Levels, regional patterns and demographic determinants, *Population Bulletin of the United Nations,* no. 25, 1988.

United Nations Secretariat, Symposium on health and mortality, *Population Newsletter,* 1997.

United Nations Secretariat, *World Health Statistics Annual 1995.*

United Nations Statistical Year Book 1996.

Verbrugge, Lois M. Gender and health: An update on hypotheses and evidence, *Journal of Health and Social Behavior,* vol. 26, no. 3, 1985.

Verbrugge, Lois M., The twain meet: Empirical explanations of sex differences in health and mortality, in *Gender, Health, and Longevity, Multidisciplinary Perspectives,* Marcia G. Ory and H.R. Warner, eds., New York: Springer Publishing, 1990.

Waldron, Ingrid, What do we know about causes of sex differences in mortality? A review of the literature, *Population Bulletin of the United Nations,* no. 18, 1985.

Waldron, Ingrid, Sex differences in human mortality: The role of genetic factors, *Social Science and Medicine,* vol. 17, no. 6, 1983.

Weiler, Paul C., *Protecting the Worker from Disability: Challenges for the Eighties,* report submitted to Minister of Labour, 1983.

Weksler, Marc E., A possible role for the immune system in the gender-longevity differential, in *Gender, Health, and Longevity, Multidisciplinary Perspectives,* Marcia G. Ory and H.R. Warner, eds., New York: Springer Publishing, 1990.

Wigle, D.T. and Y. Mao, *Mortality by Income Level in Urban Canada,* Health and Welfare Canada, 1980.

Wilkins, R. et al., Change in mortality by income in urban Canada 1971-1986, *Health Reports 1989.*

Wilkins, Kathryn, Causes of death: How the sexes differ, *Health Reports,* vol. 7, no. 2, 1995.

Wilkinson, R.G. Income distribution and life expectancy, *British Medical Journal*, vol. 304, 1992.

Wilkinson, R.G., Income and mortality, in *Class and Health*, ed. R.G. Wilkinson, London: Tavistock Publications, 1986.

Williams, A.F. and A.K. Lund, Seat belt use laws and occupant crash protection in the United States, *American Journal of Public Health*, vol. 76, no. 12, 1986.

Wingard, Deborah L., The sex differential: Morbidity, mortality, and lifestyle, *Annual Review of Public Health*, vol. 5, 1984.

World Health Organization, *Summary: The Global Burden of Disease*, C.J.L. Murray and A.D. Lopez, eds., 1996.

World Health Organization, *The Global Burden of Disease*, C.J.L. Murray and A.D.Lopez, eds., 1996.

World Health Organization, Social and economic differentials in mortality in developed countries, in *World Population Trends and Policies*, 1987 Monitoring Report.

Wyke, Sally and Graeme Ford, Competing explanations for associations between marital status and health, *Social Science and Medicine*, vol. 34, no. 5, 1992.

Yassi, Annalee, *Occupational Disease and Workers' Compensation in Ontario*, report prepared for the study of Workers' Compensation in Ontario, 1983.

Yates, J. Frank, *Risk-Taking Behavior*, Chichester: John Wiley and Sons, 1991.

Zick, C.D. and K.R. Smith, Marital transitions, poverty, and gender differences in mortality, *Journal of Marriage and the Family*, vol. 53, 1991.

Index

A
Accidents, 66, 77, 121
  automobile, 73-75, 93, 105, 107, 111, 118-19
  drowning, 75
  falls, 75
  gender, 18, 19, 73, 75, 107-108, 111
  statistics, 18, 19, 72-76, 82, 93, 105, 107, 111
  suffocation, 75. See also Alcohol, accidents
Adams, John, 77
Addiction, 67-68
Adrenaline, 27-29, 36, 38
Aggression, 30, 71, 82, 88
AIDS
  gender, 120
  spread, 120, 121-22
Alcohol, 64
  accidents, 74-75, 110-12
  benefits, 111
  disease. See Liver disease
  drinking habits, 75
  gender, 30, 37, 42-43, 46, 66-68, 72, 105, 110-12
  statistics, 53, 54, 59-60, 66, 73-75
Alzheimer's disease, 123
Androgen, 23, 30
Anti-oxidants, 55
Asbestos, 51-52
Asthma, 63, 108
Atherosclerosis, 33-34
  plaque, 33-34, 36
Automobile, 117-18. See also Accidents, automobile

B
Bronchitis, 61, 62, 108, 121
Bronze Age, 14
Brownell, Blaine, 118

C
Cancer, 77, 121, 123
  bladder, 51
  cancer process, 48-49, 50-54
  colon, 55, 114
  diet, 54-55
  esophagus, 53
  gender, 18, 19, 45-57, 88, 93, 108, 121
  lung, 49-50, 60, 63, 76, 88, 108, 110, 111, 121
  occupational, 51-52
  statistics, 18, 19, 51, 52, 53, 54, 55, 63, 64, 66, 73, 88, 93, 105, 108, 114
  stomach, 55, 114
  throat, 53-54
Cardiovascular disease. See Heart disease
Catecholamine, 36, 38, 39, 40
Cholesterol, 22-23, 28, 34, 42, 117
  types, 22-23
Chromosomes, 25, 26
Cirrhosis, 65, 77, 83
  statistics, 66, 67, 82
Cochran, Thomas, 118
Cortisol, 27
Cro-Magnon man, 14

D
Death. See Mortality
Demographic revolution, 15
Deoxyribonucleic acid (DNA), 48-49, 50, 122
Diabetes, 123-24
Diphtheria, 115
Diseases. See Gender differences
DNA. See Deoxyribonucleic acid

E
Economic implications. See Income, importance
Emphysema, 61, 62, 108, 121
Estrogen, 22, 23, 28

F
Females. See Women
Forbes, William, 80, 86, 89

142 / Why Women Bury Men

G
Galbraith, John, 125
Gender differences, 11-12
  behaviour, 18, 82-83, 116
  biology, 13-14, 17, 19, 20-32
  body weight, 56-57, 72
  diet, 41-42, 56-57, 105, 112
  exercise, 41-42
  hormones, 22-25, 36, 38
  human genome, 26-27, 123
  human immune function, 24-25
  reproductive roles, 29-30.
    See also Accidents, gender; AIDS, gender; Alcohol, gender; Cancer, gender; Heart disease, gender; Income, importance; Liver disease, gender; Men; Respiratory disease, gender; Risk-taking, gender; Smoking, gender; Stress, gender; Suicide, gender; Urban mortality, gender; Women
Gender gap. *See* Gender differences

H
Health Canada, 64, 86, 89
Health Report (Statistics Canada), 112
Heart disease, 77
  gender, 18, 19, 22-23, 25, 28, 33-43, 48, 88, 93, 106-7, 110, 111, 113, 114
  historical, 106-7
  process, 33-34
  statistics, 18, 19, 56, 59-60, 73, 76, 88, 93, 104, 112, 113, 114
Hepatitis B, 65, 66
Hirdes, John, 80, 86, 89
HIV. *See* AIDS
Hormonal replacement therapy, 23
Hormones. *See* Gender differences
Human genome. *See* Gender differences
Human immune function. *See* Gender differences
Hutton, Samuel, 46
Hypertension, 28-29, 42

I
Immunoglobulin, 24-25, 31
Income, importance, 11, 13, 16, 83, 84, 86-89, 117
Influenza, 64, 110, 119
Iron Age, 14

K
Koch, Robert, 115

L
Lancet, The, 60
Life expectancy. *See* Gender differences; Mortality
Lifespan. *See* Gender differences; Mortality
Lifestyle. *See* Gender differences; Mortality
Liver disease, 64-66
  gender, 66
  process, 65, 66. *See also* Cirrhosis
Longevity gap. *See* Mortality, longevity gap

M
Males. *See* Men
Marriage. *See* Mortality, marital status
Men, 11-13, 90
  aging pattern-shift, 16-17
  post-retirement death, 11, 93-94. *See also* Gender differences
Menopause, 23, 28, 31
Middle Ages, 14
Mortality, 18-19, 22-43
  Canadian, 11-12, 17, 22, 63, 66, 86, 90-91, 106-10, 111, 112
  childbirth, 104
  climate change, 124
  disease. *See* Gender differences
  food processing, 116-17
  gender. *See* Gender differences
  historical, 15, 17, 45, 56, 106
  lifestyle, 11-12, 17. *See also* Gender differences
  longevity gap, 18-19, 37
  marital status, 79-83, 89
  modern trends, 16, 17, 39, 45-48, 55, 56, 59, 63, 71, 75, 76, 103, 109, 118-19
  mortality rates, 15, 20, 22, 30, 37, 43, 47, 56-59, 61, 63, 81, 85, 86, 90-91, 103
  Native Canadians, 86
  pre-history, 14-15
  projections, 120-25
  science findings, 14, 103
  social class, 11, 79, 84-91
  statistics, 82, 84-86, 90-91, 93, 94, 106, 108, 113
  unemployment, 13
  urban, 91
  world, 11, 54, 56-57, 59, 66, 76, 83, 85-86, 90, 103, 104, 105, 118-19, 121, 124
Mortality rates. *See* Mortality, rates
Mortality transitions. *See* United Nations, mortality transitions